Christina Ann Morris-
Màrer tang
an leabhar beag !
le de
- ...cucha

Air Ambulance
Six Decades of the Scottish Air Ambulance Service

Iaue 2
16.1.96

Iain Hutchison

© Iain Hutchison 1996 See p. 45

British Library Cataloguing in Publication Data
Hutchison, Iain
Air Ambulance: Six Decades of the Scottish Air Ambulance Service
1. Scottish Air Ambulance Service -- History
2. Airplane ambulances — Scotland — History
I. Title.
362.1'88'09411
ISBN 0 9518958 1 8 (Softback)   ISBN 0 9518958 2 6 (Hardback)

Published by
Kea Publishing
14 Flures Crescent, Erskine, Renfrewshire, PA8 7DJ, Scotland

Phototypeset by Essprint Ltd, Stornoway
Printed by Essprint Ltd, Stornoway and Nevisprint Ltd, Fort William

In memory of my father-in-law

Prakan Premanond

Born Nakhon Sawan, 12 February 1907

Died Bangkok, 3 September 1993

ด้วยความระลึกถึงคุณพ่อ
ปราการ เปรมานนท์
ชาตะ นครสวรรค์ ๑๒ กุมภาพันธ์ ๒๔๕๐
มรณะ กรุงเทพฯ ๓ กันยายน ๒๕๓๖

Contents

Appendices

Maps

Introduction

Captain Ken Foster, Operations Director of Loganair from 1963 until 1983, gave me immeasurable help and assistance in the compilation of my first book, *The Story of Loganair*.

However I recall him taking me to task when we were reviewing the chapter on the Scottish Air Ambulance Service. My draft had made more than one reference to air ambulance flights as 'mercy missions'. Captain Foster quite rightly disapproved of my melodramatic description of this aspect of Loganair's activities.

The image which this might create, of dare-devil pilots in frail aircraft taking chances against the elements, was not compatible with modern air operations, even in the field of air ambulance flying. The truth of the matter was that most air ambulance flights were of a mundane nature, ferrying hospital patients to routine treatment on the Scottish mainland. Their flights had been arranged some time in advance and were programmed in as part of the day's regular flying programme.

Aircraft being scrambled at short notice to collect the victim of some serious accident in a remote part of Scotland were the exceptions rather than the rule. The occurrence of such flights during marginal weather conditions, which might require decisions to be taken 'at the pilot's discretion', were even more rare.

But that is not to say there has not been drama during the six decades of air ambulance flying in Scotland, operated by the early independent airlines in the days before the National Health Service, then by British European Airways and Loganair, and now shared between operators of both fixed-wing aircraft and helicopters. *Air Ambulance* recalls some of the more exciting moments of the Scottish Air Ambulance Service. But such events are small in number when weighed against the many hundreds of flights which now take place annually and which are as routine as an urban road journey.

While Part One of this book traces the development of the Scottish Air Ambulance Service, Part Two recalls some of the events that have become special memories, such as the tragic crash of a Heron on Islay which had such a profound effect on so many people connected with the service. It also frequently refers to the little touches, such as beach landings on Barra or the famous Macleod picnic basket, which have become a part of air ambulance folklore.

The account which follows is offered as a tribute to all those men and women, pilots and nurses, doctors and aircraft engineers, operations staff and ground staff, who have dedicated themselves to a service which brings greater security to Scotland's remoter communities in times of illness or accident. Even patients whose ambulance flights have been the most ordinary of aerial bus journeys extend their gratitude to them.

Iain Hutchison

Air Ambulance —

Ambulance / SAR Bases

Ⓗ Helicopter Base
✕ Fixed-wing Aircraft Base

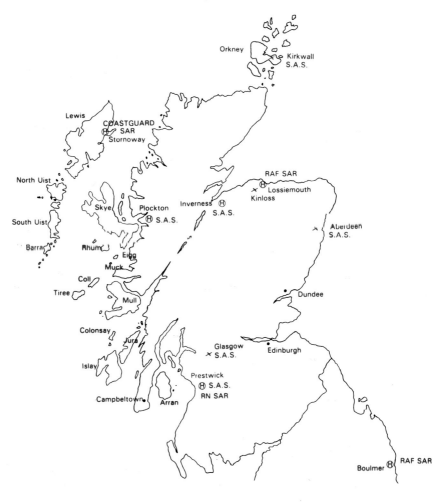

Foreword

by R E G Davies FRAeS FRSA
Curator of Air Transport, National Air and Space Museum, Smithsonian Institution

Any geographer will confirm that about three-quarters of the entire population of Scotland is concentrated in the Lowlands between the Firths of Clyde and Forth, including the cities of Glasgow and Edinburgh. Except for this area and the cities of Dundee and Aberdeen, both on the east coast, most of this mountainous country is relatively sparsely populated. The only centre of any consequence northwest of a line from Greenock to Aberdeen is Inverness which, with a population of barely 50,000, is almost a metropolis by local standards.

Cold statistics apart, any visitor to the Highlands and Islands, an area that encompasses the Grampian Mountains, the North West Highlands, the Inner and Outer Hebrides, the Orkney Islands, and the Shetland Islands, cannot but be impressed by the absence of people and the rarity of signs of habitation that characterise — and in fact enhance — the outstanding grandeur of this beautiful land.

The traveller will also quickly perceive that, in keeping with the modest transport needs of an area that is not only the most sparsely populated area of the British Isles, but also of the whole of Europe, there are not many roads — and many of these, especially in the west, are narrow, and until recently could only accommodate one-way traffic. As for railways, these are few and far between, with frequency of trains kept to a bare minimum necessary for a few essential services, and, during the season, for tourists.

All this is fine for those who go hunting, shooting, and fishing; and no doubt the animals appreciate the solitude. But for the hardy inhabitants who, from time immemorial, have eked out a simple life of crofting and fishing, the lack of communications has been the cause of economic difficulty. Nevertheless, although the inability to despatch a consignment of Fair Isle sweaters from that lonely speck of land between Orkney and Shetland may have been an inconvenience, it was not disastrous. For the hardy seafarers, inheriting stamina, skills, and instincts from generations of ancestors, delays through weather may have been irritating; but the Islanders and Highlanders moved to a different pace of life in their everyday activities, compared with the industrial workers of Glasgow or the academics of Edinburgh. And so for two millenia, life has gone on, with little fundamental change in style or custom.

Such customs have been romantically portrayed by poets and artists as idyllic; but they usually omitted to mention that, while certainly Life did go on, largely because of the resilience and hardiness of the folk to whom Survival of the Fittest was more than a Darwinian theory, so too did the Grim Reaper, Death. The remoteness of the tiny communities, distributed imperceptibly on the map like tiny seeds scattered in an inhospitable and infertile landscape, brought its own problems. These were mainly of travelling time, that in times of illness and accident, could mean the difference between Life or Death itself.

In times gone by, the rugged Scots who lived in these outlandish places were of stout lineage. They lived a hard but healthy life, and — in spite of jokes to the contrary — were invariably abstemious in their diet, and conservative in their habits. They worked hard, but did not play hard, as the saying goes — there was little time or opportunity for play.

But the harshness of the environment, and the demanding nature of their daily routine, meant that inevitably there were accidents.

During past centuries transport was almost totally by sea, for the simple reason that all the habitation was by the seaside. (A close inspection of the map reveals that few communities of more than a dozen or more souls were more than a few hundred yards from the shore.) And therein lay the problem, in some cases an insuperable one. The fastest boat could not bring an accident victim to a doctor, much less a hospital, in time to perform an operation, much less to mend a broken bone. The danger of infection was not only present, it was prolonged; and often exacerbated by the trials and tribulations of the voyage itself. Hundreds, possibly thousands of good folk died for want of medicine or medical aid that can today be purchased from any chemist.

Into this forbidding environment, in the early 1930s, came the aeroplane. Suddenly, the entire pattern of casualty evacuation underwent a metamorphosis. The balance of forces between life and death was irreversibly changed, to the eternal benefit of the scattered fishing villages and hamlets of the entire west of Scotland. Certainly, the transition did not come easily or quickly. It did not come with the advent of air transport during the 1920s. During the formative years of the airlines, aircraft were with some cause considered to be unreliable to the extent that even a slow-moving ship was a better risk than a fast-moving aeroplane that, moreover, had a worse chance than the boat of arriving at its destination and furthermore, was a riskier enterprise in the first place. For the 1920s was a period in which aircraft were used for sporting or military purposes, and were considered with much reservation as an efficient form of transport. And Great Britain's priorities for air transport did not include the development of air networks within the British Isles — a policy that was consistent with the view that the railways did a more than adequate job. Even in the 1930s, when railway-controlled, or associated independent airlines, did establish domestic networks that were neglected by Britain's flag airline, Imperial Airways, these did not reach north of Glasgow.

Such apathy to opening up the poorly-served areas of the British Isles by airline routes, to supplement the few railways, was to end in the early 1930s when a change in government regulations permitted the establishment of independent airlines. Oddly, this also coincided with another piece of legislation that abolished scores of small entrepreneur bus and coach operators to form a regulated national system. And there were several examples of the two administrative acts leading to the formation of enterprising airlines, both in England (Hillman Airways and Jersey Airways) and, more particularly, in Scotland.

Thus, in a watershed year, 1933, two airlines were formed to reach out beyond Glasgow into the Highlands and the Islands. Midland & Scottish Air Ferries was founded by a bus operator, John Sword; and Highland Airways was founded by Edmund Fresson. And a year later, another enterprising pioneer, Eric Gandar Dower, founded Aberdeen Airways. Small airfields were built in Kintyre and the Hebrides; and at Inverness, Thurso, Wick, Kirkwall and Sumburgh. Additionally, some primitive strips were cleared elsewhere, in the heather, the bogs and on the beaches, so that aircraft could land in an emergency.

While the main objective of these innovators was to inaugurate regular air services, another, humanitarian, use for the transport aeroplane was immediately realised. The evacuation of the injured or the infirm from places that lacked medical expertise to places where there were doctors (or conversely, taking the doctors to the patients) was realised to be a practicable possibility. Furthermore an aircraft could just as easily, and with little more travel time, take the patient not only to a doctor located in a nearby town, but to an airfield in one of Scotland's few cities, only a short ambulance ride from a hospital.

To state that, on 14th May 1933, Midland & Scottish Air Ferries revolutionised medical practice in Scotland when it flew an air ambulance patient from Islay to Renfrew (and who thence went by road ambulance to a Glasgow hospital) is no exaggeration. The normally conservative medical profession recognised the demonstrated advantages of an air ambulance service with little hesitation. The airline operators modified their aircraft, refined their flying techniques, and fashioned operational methods to improve beyond all recognition the speed and efficiency with which illnesses could be shortened or terminated, injuries could be healed, and lives could be saved. In Scottish medical history, renowned in other fields, this was a Red Letter Day.

The aeroplanes also brought another boon to the welfare of the islanders. Hitherto expectant mothers were either left to their own devices; or, at best, looked after by midwives when their time had come to give birth. For normal births, this was acceptable. But for abnormal circumstances, when greater skills and medical assistance were required, the happy event too often became a tragedy; and incidence of stillborn children, or, the death in childbirth of the mother, or even worse, of both, were unhappily all too frequent.

The problem was that the time between the estimated onset of labour and the estimated time of delivery was all too short — too short to take the risk of the actual birth taking place on a boat that, in the heavy swells of the western sea lanes, not to mention unpredictable storms and bad weather, would only add to the hazards, rather than mitigate them. But the speed of the aeroplane transformed the whole process. An expectant mother now stood a chance of reaching a maternity ward in a well-equipped hospital within a few short hours of the alarm call going out. And while an hour or so of possible air sickness was also likely, this was preferable to several hours of imminent sea-sickness.

If the advent of an air ambulance system may have been unnecessarily delayed — the first services in 1933 came fourteen years after regular flights were being made across the English Channel — some consideration must be given to the geographic, climatic, and demographic background and the historical development of air transport in general, both in the technical and the commercial context. Scotland had few airfields before the early 1930s — Eric Gandar Dower had to build his base at Aberdeen almost literally with his own bare hands. The low density of population raised basic economic questions about financing and support. The Hebrides and West Highlands of Scotland experience some of the highest rainfall in Europe. And — let us face it — in the early years, aeroplanes were regarded, if not actually as dangerous, as at least a hazard to a patient who was already suffering from an illness or an injury.

But having once bitten the bullet, so to speak, with the splendid initiative of the early airline pioneers, the Scottish Air Ambulance Service went from strength to strength. It grew lustily during the latter 1930s, and although handicapped in some respects during the Second World War, it benefited in others, notably by the provision of more and better airfield construction and the vast improvement in radio and telephone links that became a wartime priority. But for the War, the airports at Benbecula and Stornoway might still be grass strips.

After various changes in management, responsibility, and corporate structure, the Scottish Air Ambulance Service is an integral component of Britain's National Health Service. This latter has survived all the pressures of free enterprise advocates as a lasting tribute to the wisdom of the Beveridge Report of wartime years, and of the dedication of the postwar government of Clement Attlee and his brilliant Minister of Health, Aneurin Bevan, in seeing it through. Thanks to a truly humanitarian interpretation of the objectives of democratic socialism, the Scottish Air Ambulance Service stands as a shining example of Man's Humanity to Man — as opposed to the all-too-frequent examples of the opposite case.

Little recognition has hitherto been given to the achievements of this fine service. Anniversaries of the epoch-making flight of 14th May 1933 passed almost unnoticed by all except those intimately associated with the day-to-day running of the system. Acts of true valour and bravery, by pilots, nurses, and doctors, as they saved hundreds of lives and brought comfort and relief to thousands, were noted, if at all, only in local newspapers, and only on a few occasions were the SAAS participants awarded the testimonies they deserved.

Iain Hutchison's book, therefore, comes as a most welcome and long-awaited tribute to those men and women who contrived to create a social service of outstanding value to the people of Scotland. The narrative is painstakingly accurate, resulting from years of meticulous research. It mixes factual reporting with social commentary to provide the reader with a finely-drawn impression of the conditions under which the SAAS was able to grow to the level of praiseworthy efficiency with which the helicopters operate today. Above all, he tells the story by frequent insertions of accounts told in the words of the participants themselves, thus adding an element of what is known in academic circles as prime source material, and heightening the awareness of the reader to what was really going on.

As in his previous books, Iain echoes my own inclinations in the structural framework of his work. He provides, where appropriate, supplementary chapters that are self-contained first-hand reports by some of the veterans of the Service; there is an Appendix or two to provide technical details of the versatile aircraft on whose reliability the service depended; his maps, essential for a full grasp of the local geography, are informative and finely drawn; and he has kept the use of footnotes — too often an irritating interruption of enjoyable reading — to a merciful minimum.

Iain Hutchison's book is long overdue, but is now most welcome and should be on every library shelf. It should be read by all those who regard the aeroplane as a means of enhancing and improving our way of life, rather than as a means of destroying it. I compliment Iain for his diligence in fulfilling a heartfelt need, thank him for enriching the annals of aviation experience, and paying tribute to the exploits and achievements of the wonderful men and women of the Scottish Air Ambulance Service whose light has hitherto been hidden under the proverbial bushel.

Ron Davies
Washington DC

Jimmy and the Dragon

The first air ambulance flights performed by Midland and Scottish Air Ferries

*A*IR TRAVEL was exciting in the 1930s. Aircraft were exciting too, flimsy structures consisting of canvas stretched over wooden frames, and held aloft by two parallel pairs of wings rigged with taught wiring. They attracted thousands of spectators at the frequent air displays that were all the rage during the period between the two World Wars.

During the same era the islands of Scotland were still remote to the vast majority of the Scottish population. The fishermen who fished the waters surrounding them were hardy seafarers who regularly risked their lives as they battled their small boats against the implacable elements.

Combine the thrill of the air and those brave young men who defied gravity with the wild temperament of the Atlantic and the hardy mariners who sought to tame it. Add a life in danger, bring these two rugged types together and you have all the ingredients for some nail-biting adventure. Yet that dramatic combination passed almost without notice when they resulted in Scotland's first air ambulance flight on 14th May 1933.

The birth of the Scottish Air Ambulance Service was given bold headlines in the *Scottish Daily Express* and *The Bulletin*, but there was no great fuss on the part of the *Glasgow Herald* which, in the next day's edition, presented its account tucked away between other items of every day occurrences:

Aeroplane dash from Islay

Man rushed to hospital

A dash by aeroplane from Renfrew to Islay in order to convey a sick man from the island to the Western Infirmary, Glasgow, was made yesterday. Shortly after 9.30am a telegram was received at the headquarters of the St. Andrew's Ambulance Association asking that a 'plane be sent for an urgent case. The Scottish Flying Club were communicated with, and they in turn got in touch with Midland and Scottish Air Ferries at Renfrew.

A 'plane was immediately despatched and arrived at Bridgend 40 minutes after leaving Renfrew. The patient — John McDermid (33), fisherman, Bruichladdich — was got into the machine, which returned to Renfrew, where an ambulance waggon was waiting. He was conveyed to the infirmary, where he underwent an operation for abdominal trouble.

The patient, it is learned, is now making satisfactory progress.

Normally the patient would have taken the best part of a day to come to Glasgow by the customary boat and motor or train services.

The reporter had some doubts as to whether in fact John McDermid was the first person to be taken to hospital by an aircraft sent specifically for the purpose. However no other claims have been reported during the intervening years and his flight has remained in the history of Scottish civil aviation as the one that pioneered what was to become a regular lifeline to the islands and distant parts of the Scottish mainland.

The role that an aircraft could play in instances of such urgency was not lost on the *Glasgow Herald* which also recalled an earlier incident as a postscript to John McDermid's story:

Previous Errand of Mercy

While the flight is thought to be the first in Scotland on which a patient has been brought from an outlying part of the country to the city for an urgent operation, it is not the first time that a Renfrew 'plane has been used on an errand of mercy. Last year an aeroplane was sent off one afternoon from Glasgow to Islay carrying certain medical preparations which were urgently needed for a case on the island. As on this last occasion the journey was made in a very short space of time and without mishap.

The 'previous errand of mercy' referred to an Avro 504N from the City of Glasgow Bombing Squadron which delivered medicine from Renfrew to Port Charlotte, Islay, on 1st August 1930, not one, but nearly three years previously. This epic had begun with a telegram from Dr Stewart to the head office of Cockburn's chemists in Howard Street, Glasgow, requesting a particular medicine and intimating that it would be needed within 'a few hours'. Mr Mollison of Cockburn's started work on the prescription while his co-director, Mr Cooper, considered the merits of chartering an aeroplane. Cooper's first call was to the *Evening Times* newspaper which quickly advised him how to proceed.

Cooper first endeavoured to make contact with the Scottish Flying Club at Renfrew but met with no success. The Club was closed as it was a holiday period. But he then got in touch with Flight-Lieutenant J Whitford RAF, the adjutant of the City of Glasgow Bombing Squadron, who was happy to put an aircraft at his disposal. The medicine was despatched to the aerodrome and passed to Flying Officer Powell. Three-quarters of an hour after the plane had set off from Renfrew, the pilot was handing the vital medicine to Dr Stewart at Port Charlotte.

At 5.00pm Cockburn's received a second telegram confirming that the medicine had been received. And at 7.00pm the Avro bi-plane arrived safely back at Renfrew. It was estimated that the use of the aircraft had saved twenty-four hours, and the life of the patient.

When the first patient was airlifted three years later, it may have seemed that Dr Stewart of Bruichladdich had sent his telegram to the St Andrew's Ambulance Association on spur-of-the-moment intuition. However two de Havilland Dragon aircraft had been delivered only the previous day from the manufacturers at Stag Lane, Edgware, to go into service with John Sword's Midland & Scottish Air Ferries. And they had arrived specially fitted to carry stretcher cases and ambulance patients on the instructions of Sword who foresaw an opportunity for his new airline to provide an additional service in the very role that Dr Stewart was now requesting.

Even Sword could probably not have anticipated one of his new aircraft being pressed into ambulance duties quite so promptly. It may seem strange that the St Andrew's Ambulance Association sought to satisfy Dr Stewart's request through the Scottish Flying Club. But Midland & Scottish Air Ferries had only just launched Scotland's very first scheduled air service a few weeks earlier. Airlines in Scotland were a totally new concept.

In contrast, the Scottish Flying Club was a well-established organisation which at that time also operated Renfrew Aerodrome and from which Midland & Scottish rented its hangar space. Dr Stewart was probably also familiar with Mr Cooper's efforts to contact the flying club for assistance three years earlier.

Jimmy Orrell, who was to becom Sword's longest-serving pilot, took off for Islay in Dragon G-ACCZ at 10.25am, and at 11.15am he landed on the beach at the head of Loch Indaal, a location that he had surveyed as a landing site less than two weeks earlier, on 1st May 1933. Mrs A W Ferguson, a Glasgow nurse who happened to be spending a holiday on Islay at the time, joined Jimmy Orrell for the flight back to Glasgow to tend the ailing John McDermid. Mrs Ferguson therefore began the tradition of inflight nursing care for air ambulance patients right from the start.

Events moved on quickly, Orrell taking to the air once more at 12.20pm for a return flight of only 40 minutes. By 1.30pm McDermid was being admitted to the Western Infirmary for immediate despatch to the operating theatre. On 8th June he returned home, having overcome his ordeal, thanks to the speed of Orrell's airlift.

Ironically John McDermid's dash from Islay to Glasgow to undergo emergency treatment for perforation of the stomach, and so prevent the onset of peritonitis, was given greater news coverage in 1973.

Fully recovered from his operation of forty years earlier, McDermid was invited on a regular flight from Islay to Glasgow as a special guest of British Airways to join another local VIP on the return journey to Glenegedale aerodrome. The second guest was fellow islander Mrs Ann Heads who was returning home after having a baby and becoming the ten thousandth patient to benefit from the air ambulance service.

The now elderly fisherman was given celebrity status as he, the first air ambulance patient, was photographed with Mrs Heads as she cradled Islay's youngest resident in her arms.

While the city press in 1933 might have been slow to attach any great significance to the transfer by air of a patient needing specialist medical treatment from an outlying area to one of the city hospitals, the islanders and their general practitioners were not. No longer did the isolation of island living have to be perilous, in times of illness or accident, because of remoteness from adequate hospital facilities.

Indeed one far-sighted medical practitioner, Dr Campbell McIntyre of Port Ellen, Islay, had argued the case for air ambulances as early as 1929. 'There was much controversy during that year about a proposed hospital on Islay and I held the view that the transportation of acute surgical cases by an air ambulance was the correct procedure, a view also held by Dr Guy, then the Assistant County Medical Officer. Our views were scorned by the Department of Health and County Medical Officer but we were later able to prove to them, with the co-operation of the Scottish airlines, not only that our scheme was feasible but it was ideal. A complete change of attitude then took place and the Department and County co-operated in the scheme which was to develop.'

The feasibility of just such a scheme quickly became apparent as Renfrew-based Midland & Scottish Air Ferries found their services being called upon to provide air ambulance flights with growing frequency.

West Scotland

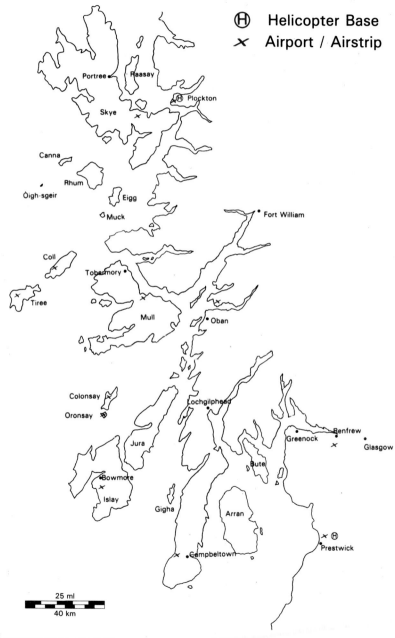

Ⓗ	Helicopter Base
✗	Airport / Airstrip

While John McDermid was still recovering from his operation, Jimmy Orrell was already responding to another ambulance call. This came on 22nd May while Jimmy was taking passengers on joy rides at an air pageant at Renfrew Aerodrome. Dr Macleod of Lochmaddy, North Uist, had read the newspaper account of the flight from Islay. Malcolm Gillies, a minister from the island, was terminally ill in a Glasgow hospital and was desperate to spend his remaining days at home on North Uist. His condition was such that he would be unlikely to survive a land and sea journey, but what about an aeroplane? The resourceful Dr Macleod soon had it all arranged and Orrell took off from Renfrew in the same de Havilland Dragon aircraft that had been used on the dash to Islay. One hour 40 minutes later he landed on a ford near Locheport. The flight signalled the first air ambulance to the Outer Hebrides and demonstrated the scope for aerial evacuation from hospital as well as to hospital.

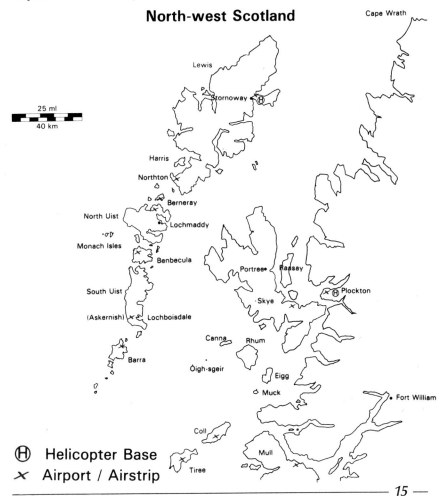

North-west Scotland

Cape Wrath

Lewis

25 ml

40 km

Stornoway

Harris

Northton

Berneray

North Uist

Lochmaddy

Monach Isles

Benbecula

Portree

Raasay

South Uist

Plockton

Skye

(Askernish)   Lochboisdale

Canna   Rhum

Barra

Òigh-sgeir

Eigg

Muck

Fort William

Coll

Ⓗ Helicopter Base

Mull

✗ Airport / Airstrip

Tiree

Captain Ed Stewart was pilot on the third air ambulance flight. This took place on the evening of 1st June with another long flight to the Outer Hebrides, this time to land in a field at Askernish on South Uist to collect an urgent medical case.

On 10th June 1933, Midland & Scottish was again called to Islay to provide an ambulance flight to Renfrew. At the request of Dr McIntyre of Bridgend, a male patient by the name of Dewar was flown out at a cost of £15. A similar flight was requested by Thomas Caskie, the airline's agent in Bowmore, three days later. Mr Caskie had been one of the two passengers who travelled on the very first scheduled flight from Islay, to Campbeltown, on 16th May.

Jimmy Orrell had been at the controls once again for these latest ambulance flights to Islay. On 14th June he then set off in Dragon G-ACCZ in search of new landing places so that access to air ambulance flights could be extended to other parts of the western seaboard of Scotland. This tour took him to Crinan, Coll, Barra, Sollas, Stornoway and Oban. Had weather not curtailed his plans, he would also have included St Kilda in his survey, although quite why is unclear because the entire population of this remote Atlantic outpost had been evacuated three years earlier.

On 19th July, Dr Alan Fothergill of Edinburgh chartered an aircraft from Midland & Scottish to fly from Renfrew to Uig on Skye, where he had taken ill while on holiday, to carry him at low altitude to Turnhouse for specialist treatment at an Edinburgh hospital. Jimmy Orrell circled over the countryside around Uig seeking a suitable spot on which to land Dragon G-ACDL. Eventually he had to settle for a risky landing up a hillside, strewn with rocks and stones, at Kilmuir. Dr Fothergill was put on board, with his wife and another doctor in attendance, and some of the stones were moved to reduce the risk of accident when the Dragon trundled down the hillside to take off again. The pilot is recorded as having navigated by the Caledonian Canal and the whole exercise was carried out during a raging storm, accompanied by thunder and lightning. The bill for this exciting journey came to £35.

On 13th September 1933, Sergeant Ronald McPhee of Govan Division Police was the charterer of an aircraft to fly from Renfrew to South Uist at a cost of £30. Upon this occasion the patient, Donald Steele, was being flown home following a sojourn in Glasgow's Western Infirmary. This time Jimmy Orrell was at the controls of Dragon G-ACCZ and accompanying Donald Steele were two sisters, and a nurse from the St Andrew's Ambulance Association. When they reached Askernish, Mr Steele had then to be carried more than a mile by stretcher to reach his home at Kildonan. The flight from Renfrew Aerodrome began at 3.00pm, with Orrell touching down again at home base five hours later.

Mr Caskie of Bowmore hired an air ambulance to fly from Renfrew to Islay on 18th September, this time on behalf of Miss Isabella McLellan of Tighan Tober, Port Ellen. The bill was for £15 'less rebate for passengers carried on outward journey to Islay' of £4. Such opportunities to subsidise the cost of an ambulance flight arose from time to time before the service was eventually financed under the National Health Service.

Statue of Edmund Fresson
at Inverness Airport with a
De Havilland Rapide in the
background during the
celebration of the sixtieth
anniversary of Highland
Airways' air mail service
to Orkney, May 1994.
(Photo by the author)

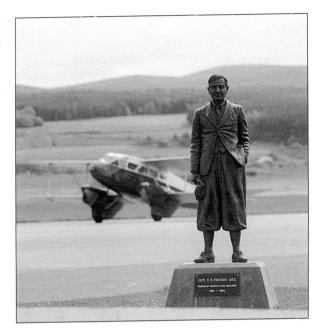

De Havilland Rapide G-ADAH of Allied Airways (Gandar Dower) Ltd.
(Photo by the author)

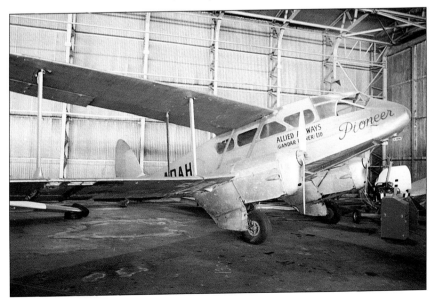

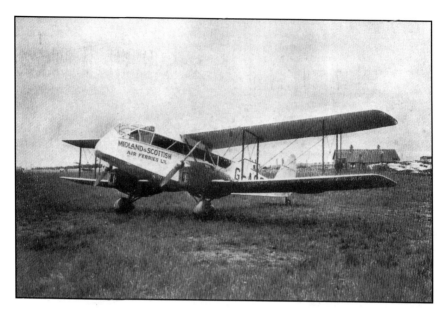

De Havilland Dragon of Midland & Scottish Air Ferries.
(Photo by courtesy of Catherine Cameron)

Captain John Rae poses before Midland & Scottish Air Ferries' de Havilland Fox Moth G-ACCU at Renfrew Aerodrome. *(Photo courtesy of Museum of Islay Life)*

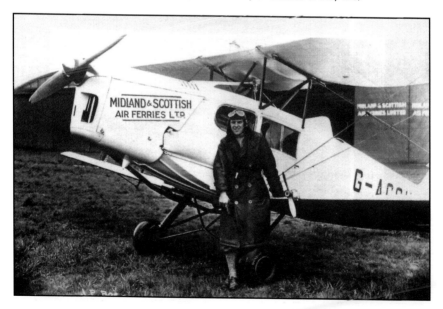

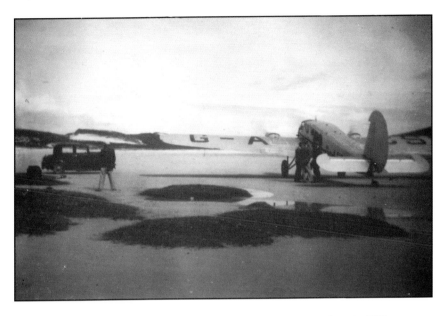

Northern & Scottish Spartan Cruiser II G-ACSM on the beach at Barra in 1937.
(Photo courtesy of Captain Ken Foster)

Northern & Scottish Spartan Cruiser III undergoing engineering checks at Renfrew.
(Photo courtesy of Bill Palmer)

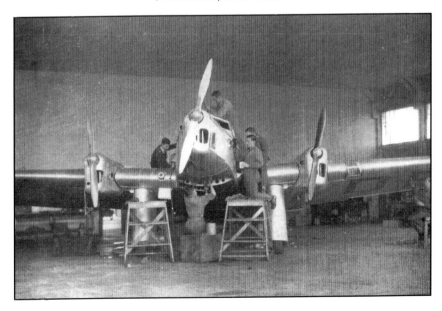

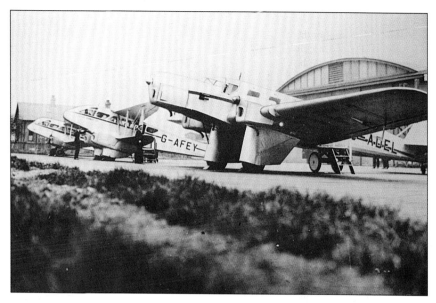

Dragon, Rapide and Spartan Cruiser III of Scottish Airways at Renfrew.

BEA Scottish Airways Heron on ambulance duty at Glasgow Airport.
(Photo by Captain Eric Starling)

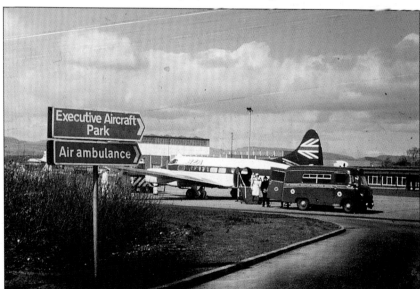

Not infrequently prospective passengers would telephone the airline's office enquiring about availability of seats after the regular scheduled service had already departed. If an empty aircraft was due out to collect an ambulance case, it would carry such passengers and the fares collected would benevolently be credited by the airline towards the cost of the ambulance charter. Miss McLellan's bill was therefore reduced to £11.

On 6th November, the Argyll peninsula was taking advantage of Midland & Scottish, on this occasion for an air ambulance charter contracted by a Mr Revie. The road route from Campbeltown is long and circuitous even now, but during the 1930s much of it was on single track roads and the route was particularly tortuous. For this reason Scotland's first scheduled air service had been inaugurated earlier in the year to link Campbeltown with Renfrew. For an invalid requiring hospital treatment, the half-hour flight to Renfrew in the hands of Captain John Rae must have seemed extremely good value at £12 10/- (£12.50) even although it represented a large sum of money for the period.

One of the more dramatic call-outs for Midland & Scottish Air Ferries had already involved Campbeltown when, on 10th October 1933, the airline was requested to send an aircraft to collect two stretcher cases. The patients, 29-year-old Stoker Henry Taylor and Stoker John Fairclough, aged 32, had sustained injuries on the Royal Navy submarine, L26, which was in the town's harbour.

A grim drama had begun two days earlier when the submarine had run aground on Paterson Rocks, one mile west of Sanda Island. The submarine, built in 1916 under the emergency war programme, lay high above the water overnight until she was refloated by the rising tide. L26 was slightly holed but she proceeded under her own power to Campbeltown Harbour for repair. But sea water had been seeping into her batteries and this resulted in a violent explosion in the harbour.

The crew had just assembled for dinner in the mess room which was immediately above the battery room. Two men, Able Seamen Leonard Rhodes and Frederick Whiting, were killed outright. They were buried in nearby Kilkerran Cemetery in a corner called Strangers Neuk where other visiting mariners had traditionally been interred. Most of the other seamen sustained serious head injuries caused by the blast throwing them directly upwards against the ceiling of the mess room. Navy personnel and local townspeople fought the blaze and fumes to rescue the injured who were transported across the harbour on fishing boats. The town had only one ambulance and many injured men were taken to the Cottage Hospital on local lorries. When it was full, those remaining were accommodated at the Poor Law Hospital.

Because of the extent and number of injuries, the Admiralty requested additional help from Professor Archibald Young, Professor of Surgery at Glasgow University. The professor set off into the night by road and reached Campbeltown at 3.00am on 10th October. He immediately set about examining the injured. Young concluded that Fairclough, suffering from a fractured thigh, and Taylor, whose left ankle had been badly crushed, needed operations at Glasgow's Western Infirmary and the air ambulance was summoned.

Fairclough seemed to be in good spirits and is recorded as turning to Jimmy Orrell as he was being carried on to the Dragon and complaining, 'I joined the Navy to go to sea, not to go on a bloody aircraft!' Taylor's condition was giving much cause for concern and he remained critical following an immediate operation at Glasgow.

The two men were accompanied by Nurse Isobel Watson of the Voluntary Aid Detachment. The charter cost £12 10/- (£12.50), plus £1 10/- (£1.50) for Miss Watson's return flight back to Campbeltown. Professor Young travelled back to Glasgow by road again that night. Thirteen men remained in hospital in Campbeltown while goodwill messages came flooding in from various well-wishers, including the naval attachés of Italy, Japan and Sweden. The L26 later made its way under escort to Devonport for repairs.

In March 1934 the St Andrew's Ambulance Association presented John Sword with 'a stretcher specially suited for air ambulance work, complete in a canvas case and weighing "only" 34lbs'. But Jimmy Orrell was not to have an opportunity to put the stretcher to use on his next call-out. On 10th April a call came in from the rugged Isle of Muck. As had been the case when he collected Dr Fothergill from Skye, Captain Orrell was once more confronted by a landscape that offered no obvious landing site and he again had to opt for an ascending run up a hillside. A safe landing accomplished, he was then informed that the locals had doubted his ability to land on the island and they had already despatched the patient to the mainland in a small boat.

As 1934 progressed, the proprietor of Midland & Scottish Air Ferries, John Sword, found himself with a dilemma. His airline pioneering was costing him a personal fortune, while he was simultaneously holding a well-paid position as General Manager of bus operators, Western SMT. The directors of SMT in Edinburgh included a powerful lobby from the railway companies who were about to set up their own airline, Railway Air Services. Sword therefore found himself with a conflict of interest and he was forced to make a painful choice. Road transport won and he started to wind down his airline from July.

However Sword was extremely conscious of the humanitarian role that the air ambulance was now playing and a Dragon aircraft (G-ACJS) was retained on standby for these duties after his other services had drawn to a close 'until another operator could be found to take it on'. During the closing months of 1934, former Midland & Scottish pilot Charles Almond, now working as an instructor for the Scottish Flying Club, was hired by Sword to perform any ambulance flight that might be required. A new operator was to appear in December in the form of another bus operator, George Nicholson.

Progress had nevertheless already taken place which would provide the service with greater financial security. In December 1933 Mr Skelton, Under-Secretary of State, announced that arrangements were being made 'to give assistance from the Highlands & Islands (Medical Service) Fund in cases of need and emergency towards the cost of the hire of aeroplanes to remove persons from the Highlands and Islands to central hospitals'. In March 1934 Skelton announced that the Department of Health had come to an arrangement with Argyll County Council under which urgent cases nominated by the local Medical Officer could be conveyed to hospital by air. Charges for the hire of the aircraft, which could not be met by the patient, would be shared by the County Council and the Department of Health.

Ambulances for the Northern Isles

*E*DMUND FRESSON'S Inverness-based Highland Airways inaugurated its first regular service on 8th May 1933. This was to Kirkwall via Wick and it forged an indelible link with Orkney that remains with Highland Airways' successors decades after that airline's passing into the realms of history and legend.

From the Orkney mainland, Fresson branched out to establish air links with several of the northern isles of Orkney. The people of North Ronaldsay enthusiastically embraced this idea and quickly got together to ensure that Fresson would not be impeded through lack of a suitable landing site. The people of Westray, Sanday, and Stronsay were soon dismantling walls to provide adequate landing runs so that they too might benefit from Highland Airways' services.

Air travel was a boon to these islands and the availability of an air ambulance service would consequently be of a special significance. This was realised in several quarters and in November, only six months after Midland & Scottish's initial ambulance flight, Fresson was operating the first ambulance flights for the Orkney Isles. This was formalised in October 1934 when he concluded an agreement with Orkney County Council for the provision of medical airlifts. The contract for the uplifting of patients from the northern isles for conveyance to the Balfour Hospital in Kirkwall came into effect immediately and was later extended to include the carriage to Aberdeen of the more serious cases requiring specialist care.

The scheme announced by Orkney County Council 'in respect of islands which have provided landing grounds' was operated in conjunction with the Department of Health which had already come to other arrangements for the Highlands & Islands and Argyll. Orkney County Council assumed the responsibility of paying the charter cost to Highland Airways which it would then recover from the patient. When a patient was unable to pay the whole cost, an affordable contribution would be agreed with the Council. Two-thirds of the remainder would then be reimbursed by the Department of Health.

Some of these early flights in the north were flown by the same John Rae who had previously flown with Midland & Scottish Air Ferries and had performed ambulance flights with Sword's pioneering airline. Rae flew with Highland Airways from 1935 until 1937 and in his first year he uplifted at least three known cases from the Orkney islands.

In his memoirs Fresson makes little reference to his own direct involvement with air ambulance flying. But he took it seriously and gave air ambulance calls the highest of priorities. These included call-outs at night for which the island airfields around Orkney were not equipped. Night landings were made possible with the aid of headlights from two motor vehicles positioned so that the beams formed a letter L across the grass. Fresson gave his pilots training at his Inverness base so that they could tackle landings on the islands with this rudimentary lighting.

The most famous of these was performed by John Hankins on 28th February 1939 when he landed on Sanday on an exceptionally dark night and during a gale. He was at the controls of one of Highland Airways' Dragons and it was considered a miracle that he found his way to the island at all. That he located and effected a landing on a 300 yard strip, helped only by illumination from the lights of a strategically parked car, was an extraordinary feat of expertise and daring. Fresson recorded, 'This flight I consider was the highlight of all our urgent ambulance flights and I have always admired the skill and courage of Captain Hankins in undertaking that call'.

Not until 9th February 1937 did any reference to air ambulance flights appear in Fresson's personal flying log. On that occasion he piloted Dragon G-ACIT to Stornoway for a landing on Melbost golf course. The patient had been in hospital in England and the 50 minute flight from Inverness, with him laid out on a specially installed mattress, would do a lot more for his well-being than the circuitous rail journey to the west coast, followed by a voyage of uncertain comfort on MacBrayne's steamer from Kyle of Lochalsh. The destination was of particular significance to Fresson as he wrote up his log. He had undoubtedly undertaken numerous earlier ambulance flights from his Orkney airfields which he would consider as routine operations not meriting special highlighting. Stornoway was different. He had long been trying to persuade the authorities on the Isle of Lewis of the benefits that would result from the construction of a proper airfield so that regular flights might be introduced. He hoped this use of his aircraft as an air ambulance would further emphasise the additional advantages that an airfield would bring them. Fresson's log records further ambulance flights to Stornoway on 30th June 1937 and 21st August 1943 but not until the closing stages of the Second World War did regular passenger flights eventually reach the Isle of Lewis.

Fresson's opposition in the north was Eric Gandar Dower's Aberdeen Airways, later renamed Allied Airways. Aberdeen Airways competed with Fresson on routes to Orkney and included an optional stop at the southern Orkney island of South Ronaldsay. Although it was later linked to the Orkney mainland by causeway, this was a useful service to the island's population in the pre-Second World War era when it was still dependent on boats. It was to South Ronaldsay that Aberdeen Airways was called to perform its first air ambulance charter on 2nd February 1936.

Eric Starling, the airline's chief pilot, set off from Thurso in Dragon G-ADFI to uplift the patient at St. Margaret's Hope, and then continue to Stromness from where the ailing man was conveyed to the Balfour Hospital in Kirkwall. Flying time from South Ronaldsay was a mere 15 minutes but Starling recorded in his log that the flight was not uneventful. 'Special ambulance run to take elderly man to Kirkwall Hospital. Owing to strong wind I took Mr Williams and Alf Cormack with me to give a hand on the ground.' The role of Williams and Cormack was to grab the wingtips and act as human anchors once the aircraft had landed and come to a halt.

Regular flights to Shetland began in 1936 and the most famous ambulance flight performed by Gandar Dower's airline, then operating as Allied Airways, occurred on 30th April 1937 when Henry Vallance was charged with the task of uplifting the keeper of the Esha Ness lighthouse from the front door of his lonely outpost in a remote corner of the Shetland mainland.

Meanwhile, on 11th November 1937, Fresson was preparing John Hankins, a pilot already enjoying a wealth of air ambulance experience gained with Northern & Scottish Airways on its Western Isles routes, for the possibility of call-outs from Fair Isle. Highland Airways and Northern & Scottish Airways had combined to form Scottish Airways on 12th August of that year and interchange of pilots was an immediate benefit of the amalgamation. Fair Isle is situated in the open sea between Orkney and Shetland. Fresson had earlier that year mastered the swirling wind eddies created by Fair Isle's sheer cliffs to land on a small piece of sloping ground which could just serve as an airstrip if its dimensions were used to the maximum by making a curved landing run.

Fresson later recalled, 'There were no downward air eddies over the approaching cliff face, but also there was no N.E. wind to help shorten the landing. Nevertheless we managed to pull up by the usual swing to the north during the middle of the landing run towards a wire fence, instead of the 200 feet cliff drop into the sea. We went up to the middle of the island with Mr Stout and a few of the islanders to settle on a site for a strip which the locals had undertaken to hew out of the hillside in their spare time. Mr Stout invited us to stay for lunch and we were served with some very tender Fair Isle mutton. The islanders were excited to see me back. We explained to Mr Stout the procedure to obtain an air ambulance flight if needed. Also, I introduced Captain Hankins, who told me he was prepared to undertake flights to Fair Isle, now that he had seen me land. I explained that Captain Hankins was in charge of Kirkwall and how to get in touch with him in case of emergency. We left for Orkney after lunch. The Dragon (G-ACIT) got off easily and I had no fear about ambulance or emergency flights being undertaken with it'. (Mr Stout was the Postmaster on Fair Isle.)

SMART WORK BY AIR AND AMBULANCE SERVICE

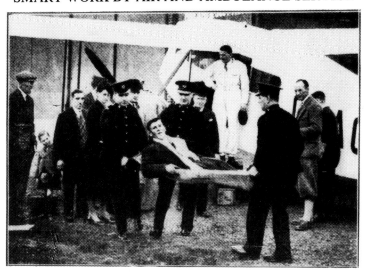

Mr John M'Dermid, an Islay fisherman, who is seriously ill and was rushed by 'plane to Glasgow for an emergency operation being carried to the waiting ambulance on arrival at Renfrew Aerodrome yesterday. Only a little over two hours had elapsed between the receiving of the S O S call in Glasgow and the patient's arrival.

Both Highland Airways and Aberdeen Airways operated de Havilland Dragons and Rapides for their scheduled services and for ambulance flights. Aberdeen Airways also used the smaller de Havilland DH80A Puss Moth for ambulance cases. The aircraft was equipped to carry only two passengers, seated one behind the other, yet was a popular aircraft for 'longer' journeys. In one instance Aberdeen Airways used its Puss Moth to fly a professor from Aberdeen to Harrogate to assist with a case of meningitis.

A flavour of Edmund Fresson's varied ambulance flying is given by the following extracts from his personal flying log.

Date	Aircraft	Winds	Time	Remarks
9 Feb 1937	Dragon G-ACIT	E	.50	Inverness-Stornoway Ambulance case. Fine. One landing.
30 Jun 1937	Rapide G-AEWL	W	1.30	Inverness-Stornoway return. 2 landings.
3 Mar 1938	Rapide G-AEWL	SW 60mph	2.10	Inverness-Kirkwall return. 2 landings.
30 Sep 1938	Rapide G-ADCT	SE	2.40	Inverness-Wick-Kirkwall-Westray return. Mail, newspapers, 3 passengers & ambulance.
25 Feb 1941	Dragon G-ACIT	—	3.15	Inverness-Orkney-N Ronaldsay-Orkney-Inverness Ambulance N Ronaldsay-Orkney. Fine. 4 landings.
6 Jul 1942	Dragon G-ACIT	E	2.35	Inverness-Orkney (Grimsetter) and return. Out Latheron owing bumps. Ambulance case. 2 landings.
5 May 1943	Rapide G-AEWL	W	2.55	Inverness-Brim Ness-Orkney (Grimsetter)-N Ronaldsay-Orkney-Inverness. Ambulance Charter.
21 Aug 1943	Rapide G-AGDG	SE	1.35	Inverness-Stornoway-Inverness. Fine, some rain on hills on return. Ambulance charter. Stretcher case.
26 Nov 1943	Rapide G-AEWL		2.00	Inverness-Sollas and return. Direct, above cloud. 18°F
26 Jul 1945	Rapide G-AGIC	N	1.15	Inverness-Benbecula. 2 patients. Blind over mountains.
26 Jul 1945	Rapide G-AGIC	N	.15	Benbecula-Barra. 2 patients & 1 passenger. Fine, some rain.
26 Jul 1945	Rapide G-AGIC	N	1.15	Barra-Inverness. 2 patients plus nurse. Above clouds.
15 Nov 1945	Rapide G-AGJG	W & SE	2.15	Inverness-Sollas-Benbecula. Direct. Used QBH.
27 May 1946	Rapide G-AGDG	NE	1.25	Inverness-Wick and return. Heavy rain, poor visibility and low cloud. 2 landings.
18 Jun 1946	Rapide G-AGDG	W	.40	Kirkwall-N Ronaldsay and return. Doctor & 2 patients.
19 Aug 1946	Dragon G-ACIT	NW	.30	Kirkwall-Stronsay and return. 4½ passengers.
22 Apr 1947	Rapide G-AGLN	S	.35	Orkney-N Ronaldsay and return. Man with crushed hand.
11 Feb 1948	Dragon G-ACIT	S	1.00	Orkney-Westray-Sanday-Orkney. Ambulance for small boy.

Behind many a dedicated ambulance pilot there is an understanding and supportive wife. Fresson enjoyed such virtues in his wife Gwen who had often been at his side throughout his pioneering activities in the air. When Edmund Fresson landed on Stronsay on 19th August 1946 to take four-year-old Barbara Cooper to the Balfour Hospital in Kirkwall with an injured leg, Gwen was on board to witness her husband's humanitarian work and no doubt also give additional reassurance to the little girl.

The Foundations of a Regular Service

Northern and Scottish Airways takes up the challenge in the West

NORTHERN AND Scottish Airways Ltd was incorporated on 21st November 1934 by George Nicholson, a Newcastle bus operator, to operate air services from Renfrew to the west of Scotland. A twice-weekly service to Campbeltown and Islay started on 1st December 1934. In January 1935 Charles Almond flew the new airline's first ambulance flight and so Northern & Scottish continued John Sword's life-saving innovation of less than two years earlier.

The airline operated initially with a fleet of de Havilland DH84 Dragons and one DH83 Fox Moth. On 23rd May 1935 Northern and Scottish came under the control of Whitehall Securities which also controlled United Airways (which incorporated Highland Airways), Spartan Air Lines, and Spartan Aircraft Ltd. This link with Spartan resulted in the addition of the Spartan Cruiser to the Northern and Scottish fleet. On 29th October a holding company was registered for the group of airlines as British Airways Ltd.

A three-engined monoplane, the Spartan Cruiser came in two variants. The Mk. II first flew in 1933. It carried two crew and six passengers and had the ugly box-shape appearance that was characteristic of several early transport aircraft. The Mk. III, which first flew in 1934, carried two crew and eight passengers. Its appearance was sleek and streamlined, in total contrast to its elder sister. The Mk. II however probably maintained a slight edge in terms of its performance.

In March 1936 David McMillan collapsed outside his shop in Campbeltown. He was diagnosed as having a perforated duodenal ulcer and the doctor gave him only four hours to live unless he was operated on immediately. The hospitals in Glasgow were five hours away by road. A telephone call was made to Renfrew only to find that the regular air ambulance aircraft was away on another flight. It was recorded that, 'A three-engined plane was rapidly transformed into an improvised ambulance and reached Campbeltown in 45 minutes'. An hour-and-a-half after his collapse Mr McMillan was being admitted to Glasgow's Western Infirmary where a successful operation was performed.

The Spartan Cruiser was often to perform air ambulance flights. On 1st June 1936 one of these machines, G-ACSM, under the command of David Barclay, became the first aircraft to touch down on the Isle of Harris.

Almost simultaneously with the arrival of the Spartan Cruisers, the de Havilland DH89 Rapide also joined the Northern & Scottish fleet. This robust successor to the Dragon was to serve in the west of Scotland for the next two decades.

Captain David Barclay, who had had a brief stint with Midland & Scottish Air Ferries in 1934 but whose flying experience extended back to 1927, made his first flight with Northern and Scottish Airways on 14th May 1935 — a local familiarisation flight in Dragon G-ACFG followed by immediate responsibility for the Renfrew-Campbeltown scheduled service. This was the beginning of a distinguished career as chief pilot with Northern and

Scottish and as an air ambulance captain whose name is still legendary throughout the Western Isles. Barclay's first ambulance case was not long in coming; he uplifted a patient from Islay in Dragon G-ACJS on 27th May. His second ambulance flight was performed a few days later when he took the same Dragon to a seldom-used landing field at Shiskine on the Isle of Arran.

In the months ahead David Barclay was to spend much time opening up airfields in the Western Isles. The prime purpose of this exercise was to develop scheduled services but it also opened the door to a growing wealth of knowledge and experience that was to be invaluable to the air ambulance service with its special demands and unique requirements in times of emergency.

One of the early landing places was Sollas on North Uist. The island had already witnessed the first air ambulance flight to the Western Isles when, on 22nd May 1933, Jimmy Orrell landed near Locheport having flown the ailing Malcolm Gillies home from the mainland. The first aircraft to land regularly at Sollas would touch down on the sands of Tràigh Ear, opposite Grenitote village, or occasionally on the silver expanse of Vallay Strand. But by 1936 aircraft were landing on a couple of strips at the southern end of Machair Leathann, near the small burial ground of Sollas village. For a time Captain John Hankins was based here and the landing site was fitted out with a hangar and a fuel pump.

John Hankins, a New Zealander, was held in high regard in North Uist as Alick Macaulay of Paiblesgarry recalls. 'He often landed on the machair which led out to Aird a' Mhòrain and he could land there from either direction. There was no windsock, but he used the marram grass to judge the wind direction. The crofters would be informed in advance of the arrival of the plane so that they could remove their cattle from the machair.'

By 1936 air ambulance flights had already settled into an established and even regular pattern. This is illustrated by a report in the *Daily Record* on Tuesday 7th July of that year.

Air Ambulance Busy — three Patients flown to Hospital

'Northern and Scottish Airways conveyed three urgent sickness cases to Glasgow yesterday — one from Campbeltown by the ordinary services and two from Lochmaddy, North Uist. A special run had to be made for the North Uist cases — Mrs McLellan, a maternity patient, and Master McDonald, admitted to the Western Infirmary, Glasgow, suffering from an internal complaint.'

'A passenger on the 'plane from Campbeltown, Mr P C Baldie of Glasgow, gave up his seat to allow Mr James Wallace to be flown to Glasgow, where he was operated on within an hour or two for appendicitis. Mr Baldie had an important business appointment in Glasgow in the afternoon. He sacrificed it on Mr Wallace's behalf.'

'The ordinary service 'plane to the Outer Hebrides had completed the round trip and was back in Renfrew when a telegram was received from Lochmaddy asking for a 'plane to convey Mrs McLellan and Master McDonald to Glasgow. The seats were stripped from a Spartan Cruiser and two stretchers installed. The machine was in the air within 15 minutes of the S.O.S being received. It was back in Renfrew before eight o'clock and the patients, who had Nurse Campbell accompanying them, were rushed to hospital in ambulance wagons.'

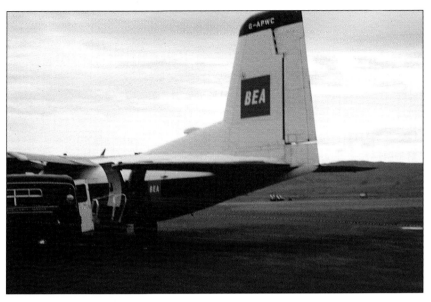

BEA Handley Page Herald on ambulance duty at Campbeltown.
(Photo by Lesley Crawford)

End of an era. BEA Scottish Airways Heron at Barra
and the short SC7 Skyliner that was to take over its scheduled service duties.
(Photo by Captain Ian Montgomery)

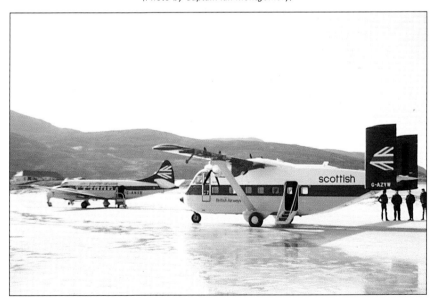

Page 4

Holder has permission to retain this Permit for repeated journeys within the dates of validity.

THIS PERMIT IS ONLY VALID WHILE THE BEARER IS IN THE EMPLOYMENT, WITHIN THE PROTECTED AREA, OF *Scottish Airways Ltd*

D.R. Form 7

N⁰ P.553794
PERMIT TO ENTER
a Protected Place or Area
as defined in the Defence Regulations

General Conditions
1. This Permit is available only to enter the Place or Area described on Page 2.
2. This Permit is issued subject to the provisions and penalties of the Defence Regulations.
3. The loss or finding of this Permit should be reported at once to the Issuing Office or to the Police. The Bearer should carry this Permit in an addressed envelope to preserve it from damage and to facilitate its restoration if mislaid.
4. This Permit must be presented on the demand of a person on duty who is a member of His Majesty's Forces, or acting on behalf of His Majesty, or a Policeman.
5. This Permit must be returned to the Issuing Office on or before date of expiry; and in the event of the Bearer ceasing to hold any appointment or occupation on account of which this Permit was issued.
6. This Permit must be supported by the production of an official Document of Identity containing a photograph of the Bearer.

Page 2

PERMIT *Jane G. Govan,*
of (address) *9, Orr Square, Paisley.*

TO ENTER NUMBER ONE AREA

for the purpose of *Duties as Nurse (Air Ambulance)*
Available from *14-6-41*
Validity expires *14-12-41*
unless withdrawn, or extended by endorsement on page 4.

Issued at MILITARY PERMIT OFFICE
On behalf of ... 19 JUN 1941
by
on /N.

Page 3

PERMIT N⁰ P.553794 G/2802 354.
Nationality of Bearer *British*

(Office Stamp)
THIS PERMIT IS ISSUED SUBJECT TO ANY ENDORSEMENTS HEREON. This Permit does not admit to any closed part or building within a Protected Place without special permission and is valid only when the Bearer produces the following Document of Identity on demand :

British Subject Identity Card No. *SNTD. 5*
British Passport No.
Aliens Registration Certificate No.
.....No.

Signature of Bearer *J.G.Govan*

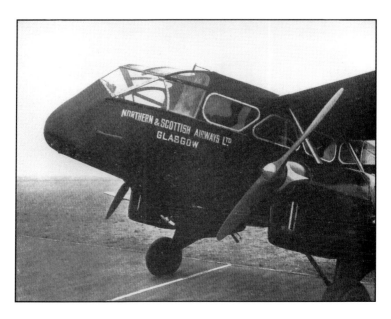

De Havilland Dragon of Northern & Scottish Airways.
(Photo courtesy of Bill Palmer)

Pilot and nurse prepare for the departure of an early BEA Rapide flight.
(Photo courtesy of Tony Naylor)

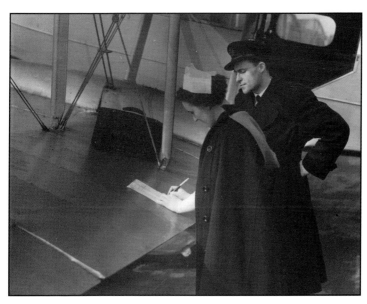

Ann Heads with her new newly born baby, the 10,000th air ambulance passenger, with John McDermid, the first patient, at Islay Airport in 1973.
(Photo BEA, courtesy of Tony Naylor)

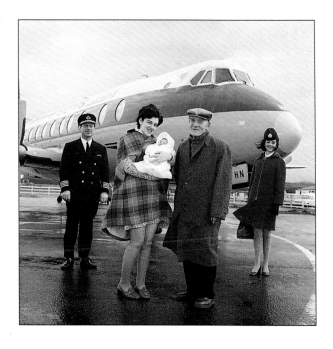

Piper Aztec G-ASYB which performed Loganair's first air ambulance flight in 1967.
(Photo by Captain Ken Foster)

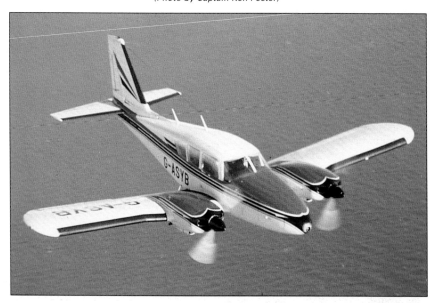

In August 1937 Northern & Scottish Airways and Highland Airways were amalgamated as Scottish Airways but still continued to operate as two distinct divisions from their respective bases at Renfrew and Inverness. From Renfrew the bulk of air ambulance flying was being undertaken with DH84 Dragon and Spartan Cruiser Mk. II equipment. The DH89 Rapide was used in this role occasionally but by early 1940 no Dragons remained in the fleet and the Spartan Cruisers were being requisitioned by the Royal Air Force. The Rapide then took over as the workhorse of the Renfrew Division of Scottish Airways.

The custom of having a medical attendant on board an ambulance flight was established from the presence of holidaying Glasgow nurse, Mrs Ferguson, on the very first such flight from Islay in May 1933. Sometimes a doctor would accompany a patient but more often the District Nurse from the island would tend the patient on the journey to the mainland.

This presented problems because the District Nurse would then have to make her own way home, usually by train or bus, followed by a sea journey. An island could therefore be without the services of its district nurse for two or even three days when an air ambulance had been summoned.

The solution was for a mainland-based nurse to fly out with the aircraft and look after the patient during the airlift from the island. In 1938 the Royal Alexandra Hospital in Paisley was approached by Dr Shearer of Edinburgh and the Medical Officer for Argyll with this proposition. However the matron would have none of it. She was not prepared to put the lives of her nurses at risk by asking them to travel in the frail aircraft.

The matron instead referred these gentlemen to two nurses, Margaret Boyd and Jean Govan, who had a private nurses association in Paisley. Margaret and Jean agreed to undertake this service which was inaugurated on 1st March 1938, and Margaret Boyd embarked on the first call-out under this new agreement on 4th March. That flight to Islay was Margaret's first taste of air travel, undertaken in perfect flying conditions, and she returned to Renfrew with her patient, a young boy suffering from appendicitis, who proceeded to Glasgow Royal Infirmary for an operation.

The DH84 Dragons and Spartan Cruisers of Scottish Airways could land in many inhospitable places but even these versatile aircraft had their limitations as a Northern & Scottish Airways 'Memorandum on the Air Ambulance Service' recalls. 'On 3rd August 1939 an urgent call was received from the island of Colonsay. As no landing facilities are available on the island, arrangements were made for the patient to be conveyed by speed-boat to Port Askaig on the island of Islay from which point the patient was conveyed by road ambulance to the Company's aerodrome at Port Ellen, and thence by Air Ambulance to the mainland where a landing was made at 11.45pm. In all, the patient's journey from Colonsay to the Western Infirmary, Glasgow, occupied less than three hours, whereas the ordinary steamer was not scheduled to call at Colonsay until the following day and a surface journey by boat and rail of upwards of 15 hours would have been entailed.'

An account of the air ambulance service, excerpted from an article by George Blake in the *Scottish Daily Express*, appeared in the Scottish Airways illustrated brochure for 1939.

'Hullo! Hullo! Hullo! Is that Renfrew 230?'

'This is Renfrew 230. Scottish Airways speaking.'

'This is Dr M------ of Tiree. I have a very urgent case for hospital. When can you let me have the Air Ambulance?'

'Right away. Can you get your patient comfortably to the Reef Airport? Good. Western Infirmary, Glasgow. Righto, doctor! Expect the plane in about an hour's time and have your patient ready.'

And within three hours that so far nameless patient in Tiree will be in an operating theatre in a highly-equipped Glasgow infirmary, safe in the care of a specialist surgeon.

Six years ago, the doctor will reflect, that life would almost certainly have been lost. A diseased appendix, a shooting accident, or a bicycle smash would have meant, at the best, a make-shift operation by a general practitioner in a rarely-used cottage hospital. In remoter parts it would probably have meant just doing the best to ease the agonies until the inevitable end came.

Now the most remote crofter of the Outer Isles has as fair a chance of speedy and expert treatment as a Lanarkshire miner.

The use of a plane for ambulance work started in 1933. The then operator of the Western Isles services was generous in giving the use of his machines to an occasional urgent case. One of the ambulance associations presented a special stretcher.

In 1935, however, the Argyll County Council entered into a regular arrangement with Northern and Scottish Airways — now Scottish Airways Limited — in connection with the Highland Medical Service under the aegis of the Health Department for Scotland. Inverness County Council followed suit.

Power to call out the air ambulance is vested in certain doctors in the Highlands and Islands Medical Service of the Health Department. Of these Scottish Airways possesses a check-list. The costs of a flight — which works out at about £10 per flying hour — are divided between the department and the county council concerned in cases where the patient is unable to contribute.

From January 1935 to January 1939 the Air Ambulance Service as officially recognised had carried some 300 cases. The vast majority of these recovered — lives saved that would almost certainly have been lost six years ago.

An ambulance call is the signal for a positive fret of activity at the Renfrew Airport. Sometimes it may be possible to pick up the patient on the ordinary service run. The pilots can show you logbook entries telling how, over the Firth of Lorne, say, they were wirelessed to divert from their course to pick up a patient dangerously ill.

In the early days, it was usually a case of bringing the district nurse back with the patient. This took invaluable public servants away from their areas, and now the practice is to send a nurse with the Air Ambulance.

Meanwhile, our pilot and wireless officer are on the airfield. The plane is being serviced according to a hard-and-fast schedule for there must be no possibility of error or mishap.

Petrol tanks are filled. The stretcher is fitted. The nurse in her blue uniform takes her seat. The wireless officer sits at his instrument waiting. The pilot climbs in.

'Contact!'

The engines, already heated by 10 minutes' free running, roar into life as the mechanics swing the propellers. Away she taxies across the field for a fair take-off into the wind. She gets the gun, as the airmen say; she rears and rises and heads nor'-west. Another race for life has started.

But they are still busy in the offices of Scottish Airways.

Somebody has arranged for a St. Andrew's surface ambulance to be waiting the plane's return. Somebody has 'phoned an E.T.A. to the anxious doctor in the isles — E.T.A. being simply expected time of arrival. Somebody has mobilised the ground staff to run out the flares if a return in darkness is expected.

At the Air Ministry Control Station, men wearing head-phones are listening to Morse messages from the ambulance, giving bearings and special weather forecasts in return. Each message is passed to the Control Officer who transmits by phone to the company. Then a great responsibility rests mainly on the pilot for a time.

Probably it is the Chief Pilot — Captain David Barclay, small, brown-faced, clear-eyed. He is wresting all the time with the dirty weather of the western seaboard.

Naturally, the air ambulance tries to pick up its helpless passengers at an organised landing-place. But sometimes the Pilot has to use a mere strip of wet beach, a runway indicated by the doctor himself, or even to discover a small field that will serve in the emergency.

Every Scottish Airways' Aerodrome has its own emergency stretcher for ambulance work. And Captain Barclay has been so long on the job that he knows every conceivable landing place from the Mull of Kintyre to the Butt of Lewis.

The air ambulance has never had a flying mishap.

Behind the pilot sits the wireless officer. The whole safety of the machine is depending as much on the quickness of his mind as on the pilot's skill.

He reports his position from time to time — over Lochgilphead, over the Ross of Mull, over Gigha — and QBG 3,000: that is, flying above cloud at 3,000 feet. And Renfrew is feeding him back, perhaps, another special weather report.

But it is only too easy to lose your bearings over the West Coast of Scotland. And Renfrew gives back at once a true bearing from that point.

If there is any doubt they give back 'a cut' — that is, two or three bearings from different wireless stations: Renfrew, Sollas in North Uist, or Newtownards in Ulster. Where the lines of the compass bearings intersect on the map before him — well, that's where he is.

They even give him barometric pressure. That affects the instrument that tells him his altitude.

Then their last signal of all from the plane — QAL. About to land. The pilot sees below him tiny dots in the grey light of dawn or the ruddy mirk of a winter sunset, the pathetic party — doctor, district nurse, relatives, and the white-faced patient he had flown perhaps 150 miles to succour. The plane banks, lands and taxies along the sand or turf, and comes to rest.

It doesn't take long nowadays to get the stretcher in. They have mastered the tricky art of edging it through a plane's narrow doorway. It is securely clamped on one side normally occupied by single seats for passengers.

'Contact.'

It has taken only five minutes. Barra — or Coll — or Tiree is a patchwork of fields far below. The Nurse is calmly taking the temperature of her new patient and explaining how simple and comfortable this flying business is, and what good doctors they have in Glasgow.

The Wireless Officer is back at his panel. The sharp rasping of the vigilant Morse signals is always in his ear. He gets a reassuring message that all is clear in the troublesome Clyde weather area and passes a chit to the Pilot.

The surface ambulance is waiting at Renfrew. There is an empty bed with aired sheets in a big Glasgow hospital. A surgeon is ready to diagnose and act.

The men in Radio Control on the airfield get through the headphones the plane's letter of identification and then a bold — — · — · — · — · · (spelling QAL in Morse) which means winding in aerial to land.

The Air Ambulance has been out and back for nearly the 300th time.

The nurse referred to would at this time have been either Margaret Boyd or her friend and colleague Jean Govan.

The same publication carries advertisements from Glasgow hospitals keen to receive air ambulance patients . . . and donations. The Western Infirmary lays out its credentials with the information that in 1938 it had treated 13,576 patients in Wards, 51,506 patients at the Dispensary and that its maintenance expendure was £113,714, treatment costing 8/- per patient per day. But Glasgow Royal Infirmary was not to be outdone in proclaiming its popularity with island patients, or at least their doctors. Its advertisement entices donations with the news that 'From the lonely sheilings and misty isles of the North and West of Scotland more than 200 patients were brought last year to the largest Voluntary Hospital in the West of Scotland'.

The bill for the hire of the aircraft for these early flights had to be borne by the patient and his family, but of course the sum involved was often quite beyond their means. As a result they might contribute what they could reasonably afford, with the remainder being provided by the local community which often established a special fund for this contingency. Sales of work, whist drives, concerts, and cèilidhs were employed to sustain these community schemes, making it possible for the financial burden involved, when serious illness or accident occurred, to be borne without bankrupting the patient and his family.

In his 93rd year, Alex Campbell recalled his time as general practitioner in the Parish of Kildonan and Oa on the Isle of Islay. 'There was no proper landing strip on the island but, to begin with, a flat grassy field on Duich Farm was used, near the roadside, about half way between Port Ellen and Bowmore. Very occasionally the beach at Bridgend, at the head of Loch Indaal, was used for landing but this depended entirely on the state of the tide. I sent one patient away from here, 56-year-old Duncan Ferguson of Ardelistry. He was suffering from appendicitis and he had never been off the island before. Request for an air ambulance was not made lightly as there was not much money about in those days and the patient was nominally responsible for the cost.'

'So far as Kildonan and Oa parish was concerned, the situation was alleviated to some extent by the action of Mr Harry Clifton, the proprietor of Kildalton Estate at that time. One day, out of the blue, he handed me a cheque for £50 to be used for any philanthropic purpose which I might think fit. I consulted the local bank manager, Mr William Aitken, and we set up a fund, called The Doctors' Fund, with that gift as a beginning. The fund was thereafter augmented by the proceeds from concerts, dances, whist drives, etc., and the occasional donation. There was never a great deal of money in the fund but usually sufficient to give much needed help to patients travelling by air ambulance, or indeed by the ordinary route involving two steamers and a train journey, because non-urgent cases continued to go by this method.'

'I have a good recollection of one of the first times I used the air ambulance in the very early days. I was called to see a patient, William Cameron, late one afternoon. I found him very ill with a perforation of the stomach. Knowing that he had a poor chance of survival if he had to wait overnight and travel by steamer next day, I made a desperate request for an air ambulance, even though I knew it would probably be dark by the time a plane could arrive. We had no telephone in Islay until the late 1930s so all urgent messages had to be sent by telegraph. However Scottish Airways and their courageous pilot 'turned up trumps' and sent a plane which we helped to make a landing on the Duich field with the aid of car headlights.'

'As the patient was only going to be accompanied by a somewhat nervous relative, I decided on the spur of the moment to accompany them myself so, after sending a message to my wife, I did just that. Having got safely off the ground, rather bumpily we arrived at Renfrew Airport about one hour later. On one occasion during the flight, on happening to glance out the side window of the plane, I saw what I took to be an exhaust glowing red hot. Being ignorant of such matters, I wondered ''Is this normal, or does it mean that we might get blown sky high before we reach our destination?'' An ambulance was awaiting our arrival at Renfrew and we were soon in the Western Infirmary, Glasgow.'

'I attended the patient's operation which went into the small hours of the following day, performed by a surgeon called Mr Maitland. After seeing my patient safely in bed I went to spend what was left of the night with relatives in Glasgow. In the morning I returned to Renfrew Airport to investigate the possibility of getting a flight back to Islay. A plane was just about ready to set off and there was one seat available but unfortunately when I was weighed I was told that I was too heavy! However Scottish Airways were more than generous as they put on another plane specially for me. I was the only passenger and the pilot wore plus-fours.'

In Campbeltown a formal ambulance scheme was set up by the Campbeltown & District Co-operative Society Ltd. This began operation on 14th January 1937 and by 15th March 1939 it was being recorded that 220 people, including attendants, had travelled as a result. 155 of these had travelled by rail and steamer, 49 by regular flights, and 16 by road or air ambulance. The report for this period indicated that the operation had cost £263 12s 6d. Income had been £341 16s 9d, leaving a balance of £78 4s 3d. The average cost of each person travelling was £1 5s 9d. The scheme in action was reported in the *Campbeltown Courier* of 1st April 1939.

'The value of the Air Ambulance service administered by Scottish Airways Ltd in association with the Campbeltown and District Co-operative Society was strikingly demonstrated on Tuesday. The Air Ambulance had only just completed an emergency run from Islay when it was required to convey a small patient, Campbell MacMaster, from Campbeltown to Glasgow for hospital treatment. Mr James MacGeachy, the Campbeltown Airport Superintendent, at once took the necessary steps to have the Air Ambulance sent back to Campbeltown with Nurse Boyd of Renfrew in charge of the transport of the case. A very quick journey was made and the little patient was rushed to hospital.'

In 1939 there were 800 members in the Campbeltown ambulance scheme, representing 75% of the Society's total membership of 1,060. Taking dependants into consideration, it was estimated that about 2,400 were eligible for its benefits. The scheme was unique and after two years of operation was creating interest throughout the country and had stimulated enquiries from abroad. The Campbeltown society joined the Scottish Co-operative Wholesale Society in 1947.

A role with financial aid was also undertaken by county councils such as those for Argyll, Inverness-shire and Orkney. The cushion which they provided must have given ever greater comfort as the hard years of the Second World War took their toll. Helen Sutton had experience of the service which operated during that time with aircraft with their windows masked so that passengers could not observe the movements and installations of the armed services.

'It was January 1943 when I was taken on an emergency air ambulance for the birth of my first baby. My husband was stationed at Forres at the time and was on leave at my parents' home at Stewarton on Kintyre. In those days the plane was using an airstrip on a field at the Strath Farm or at Dalivaddy. It was a very foggy day and the plane had to be diverted from its usual landing place but we got to Glasgow eventually.'

'It was a very distressing time for me and my family. With the war and all the restrictions, my parents couldn't even visit me in hospital and I saw no one for a fortnight. My baby did not survive and the hospital said that I was unfit to travel back to Campbeltown by road or unaccompanied. After several days my husband obtained a 48-hour pass. You can imagine how relieved I was to get a telegram from him to say he was on his way to take me home by plane. The £6 donation that we paid to Argyll County Council seems a very small pittance today.'

Although civil flying in Scotland was curtailed during the early period of the war, the continuity of air connections for the islands soon proved to be essential. This was no less true of the air ambulance service. In May 1940 Mrs Peggy McKinnon of Ardvore was Barra's first wartime case, uplifted by Captain Donald Prentice with Radio Officer Hugh Black and Nurse Boyd.

On 10th December 1940, as a direct result of the war, an air ambulance uplifted six sailors from Barra. Their ship had been torpedoed in the Atlantic and they had spent many days in an open boat before being driven ashore on the island and in desperate need of medical attention. Margaret Boyd, now 90 years of age, recalls this incident. 'It was my friend, Jean Govan, who went out with the plane to pick up these sailors. They were badly frostbitten and gangrene was setting in. The people of Barra did the best they could to help them until they were flown to Glasgow and they had given them all big heavy hand-knitten woollens. One of the sailors did not recover.'

As the Second World War advanced, increasing numbers of nurses were called up for military service. This had severe implications for the staff resources available to the Paisley Nurses Association so that by February 1942 Margaret Boyd and Jean Govan could no longer put themselves at the disposal of the air ambulance service and they relinquished their role to the Southern General Hospital. The first nurses from the Southern General had to be 24 years of age before they were permitted to fly and they included Barbara McCorkindale, Anne Wilkie, Zena McGomery, Dolly Smith and a Nurse Walker.

Anne Wilkie had made her first flight in March 1936 when she accompanied an ambulance to Sollas to uplift 13-year-old Ina McDonald. Sister Wilkie had indicated only one hour earlier that she would be a volunteer for ambulance flights and she had never previously been airborne. She was given no time to pause for second thoughts.

Barbara McCorkindale's most unusual flight was to come much later, in 1950, when she was asked to fly to New York to bring an invalid woman home to Scotland. The request came from the Foreign Office which was responsible for the patient's repatriation. Babs McCorkindale had to wait in New York for five days while her patient was brought by ambulance from Boston. Then, during the return journey, the aircraft, a BOAC Stratocruiser, had to divert from mid-Atlantic to Gander for an emergency landing after developing engine trouble. For Babs, the total operation had lasted nine days.

Scottish Airways continued its air ambulance work throughout the Second World War until it was absorbed into the British European Airways Corporation upon nationalisation of the independent airlines in 1947. But by 1943 the air ambulance service was established as a routine aspect of the airline's operations. It was reported as a slick flexible system, well tried and tested, where the air ambulance could be despatched at short notice in an emergency. 'Stretchers are retained at all Out-Stations of the Company in the Western Isles and frequently an ordinary Service Aircraft is diverted in the course of its normal Service Flight to bring urgent Ambulance cases to the Mainland and Service passengers, temporarily displaced, complete their journey by means of a relief aircraft sent out from Renfrew. On no occasion has any regular passenger made any complaint regarding delay caused by the interruption of a Regular Service to perform Air Ambulance work.'

Air Ambulance —

Between January 1935 and 31st July 1943 Scottish Airways recorded 540 ambulance flights from Renfrew to airfields in the Western Isles. In addition, it noted that numerous sitting patients had also been conveyed on its ordinary scheduled services. Ten years on from Midland & Scottish Air Ferries' dash to Islay to aid John McDermid, the Scottish Air Ambulance Service already had a proud history and reputation which would continue to provide inspiration to those who would follow in the wake of the early pilots, nurses, doctors, and patients.

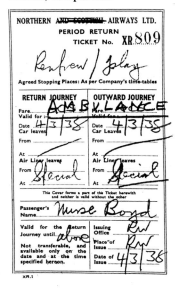

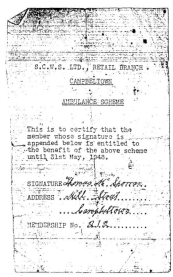

Argyll County Council,

Campbeltown., 3rd May 1943.

Dear Sir,

Air Ambulance Service

I thank you for your letter enclosing the sum of Six Pounds (£6) Stg. in payment of the proportion of the cost of the air ambulance which was ordered for Mrs. Sutton recently.

Yours faithfully,

Treasurer.

Mr.E.A. Sutton,
    Allendale,
      High Street,
        GREAT GLEN,
          Leicester.

The arrival of BEA
and the National Health Service

B RITISH EUROPEAN Airways Corporation took over the services and aircraft of Scottish Airways on 1st February 1947. Financial arrangements for ambulance flights were not immediately affected but on 5th July 1948, with the formation of the National Health Service, it was provided to patients free of charge.

BEA continued to operate the de Havilland DH89 Rapide for ambulance flying and for some of its Scottish scheduled services. The first birth to be logged in the Register of Air Births held at Register House, Edinburgh, took place in one of these. Margaret McLellan was in advanced labour when the aircraft landed at Stornoway after the short flight from Benbecula on 22nd November 1949. Another patient with a broken leg was rushed off the aircraft, and Nurse Anastasia Doherty, assisted by BEA's Stornoway agent, Mrs McPherson, completed the delivery of a baby boy. There were no facilities at the airport but the aircraft had an electric light which was the only technological aid at the nurse's disposal.

The first birth to take place in the air occurred on 28th February of the following year when Lachlan Macfarlane was born above the Gulf of Corrievrechan while his mother was being flown from Tiree to Renfrew. The Rapide, under the command of First Officer Stanley Brown, had been diverted from the Hebrides scheduled service to uplift Mrs Christina Macfarlane.

The Rapide continued faithfully in the service of BEA during the early days of the new corporation and, in its ambulance role, on 24th May 1948, it ventured as far west as Shannon, one of the rare international mercy flights. During this period David Barclay was also occasionally flying Ted Fresson's favourite Dragon, G-ACIT, using it to take Renfrew-based pilots on survey flights to Tiree, Islay, Mull, Colonsay, Oronsay, Coll, Benbecula, Sollas, and Northton (Harris) to familiarise them with regular and irregular landing sites in the Hebrides serving communities which might call on the air ambulance for assistance. Barclay also took G-ACIT to Orkney airfields on Sanday, Westray, and North Ronaldsay where the aircraft had been a familiar sight when operating for Highland Airways.

Such survey and crew training flights continued in 1948 with the Rapide. David Barclay's log for 22nd June reads, 'Grimsetter-Stronsay-Sanday-North Ronaldsay-Westray-Grimsetter. Air ambulance field training experience for Capt Rayer, Capt Hayes, F/O Harriden. Grimsetter-Aberdeen-Renfrew. Route training for F/O Harriden.'; and on 30th June, 'Renfrew-Coll-Benbecula-Northton Beach-Kirkwall-Stronsay-Sanday-North Ronaldsay-Westray-Kirkwall-Aberdeen. 7 hours 23 minutes. Air ambulance landing fields experience for Capt Appleby'.

Rapide G-AHVX landed at North Ronaldsay on an ambulance flight on 15th January 1949. The grass strip was severely waterlogged and the aircraft was badly damaged when it made contact with the ground. It was considered beyond repair and in future BEA preferred to avoid these rough strips whenever possible.

In 1953 consideration of a replacement for the Rapide biplane began and by January 1954 this was becoming a matter of urgency because no natural successor, capable of landing on the smaller airstrips and beaches, appeared to be available. An example of such a landing site was Sollas on North Uist.

Sollas airfield had been opened by Northern & Scottish Airways in 1936. Two grass runways were laid out, a hangar erected, and a fuel depot built. Sollas fell into disuse as a stop on the scheduled service of BEA with the introduction of the DC-3s. To use the air service, passengers from North Uist then had to cross to Benbecula by boat or ford the channel separating the two islands in a cart. Air ambulances would still land at Sollas but the crofters on whose land the airstrips lay were anxious to return their land to full use because visits by aircraft became an infrequent occurrence. Landings on the adjacent beach therefore became the pattern whenever the air ambulance was required to make a visit to North Uist.

When, in December 1954, the Secretary of State announced that he had agreed to the purchase of two de Havilland DH114 Heron aircraft to replace the Rapides on the Air Ambulance Service and the scheduled service to Barra, he reserved the right to ask for their replacement later by the Scottish Aviation Twin Pioneer if the latter proved to be a more suitable choice for air ambulance work. Orders for the Twin Pioneer did not materialise from BEA and this was later to be a source of some frustration to Scottish Aviation. An order from BEA would have been a useful endorsement for the manufacturer in its worldwide efforts to market its unique STOL aircraft.

During the final year of operation of the Scottish Air Ambulance Service by Rapide aircraft, the trusty biplanes were recorded as carrying 311 patients on 258 flights over a total of 59,365 miles. The last flights were performed by G-AHKS *Robert Louis Stevenson* and G-AJXB *William Gilbert Grace*. G-AHKS had flown a mere 414 hours in BEA service since January 1947 out of a total of 6,712 hours 'on the clock'. G-AJXB had been acquired in December 1948 and had 491 hours flown in BEA service out of a total of 6,428. Both aircraft were sold on 25th April 1955.

The Heron 1Bs delivered to BEA were models specially adapted with Scottish island operating conditions in mind. Called the 'Hebrides' class, the Heron's fixed nose wheel had a special guard designed to minimise salt water spraying on to the engines and propellers, an important feature for operations to such landing sites as the beaches at Barra and Sollas. During July 1954 Heron trials had taken place to these airfields and also to Harris, Coll, North Ronaldsay and Sanday.

On 18th January 1955 David Barclay undertook his initial instruction at Hatfield on the de Havilland Heron. Under the tutelage of Captain Bais of de Havilland, Barclay executed five take-offs and landings and other manoeuvres such as turns and stalls. By February BEA's first Heron had arrived at Renfrew, but Barclay's ambulance flights continued in Rapides while his Conversion Course in the Heron progressed. The first ambulance flight in a Heron (G-ANXB) took place on 4th March 1955, with Barclay seconding Captain McKenzie on a flight to Benbecula.

David Barclay completed his Conversion Course in March and the two aircraft were formally dedicated at a special ceremony at Renfrew on the 18th. The nose of each aircraft was anointed with champagne by Miss Jean Jolly, matron at the Southern General Hospital. David performed a flypast at the ceremony in Rapide G-AHKS.

The introduction of the Heron was a gradual process which continued well into April, Barclay now acting as instructor to other pilots flying from Renfrew. Ambulance call-outs continued to be performed with the familiar Rapide until Barclay took Heron G-ANXA on an ambulance flight to Barra on 28th April. Over the next few days he flew Herons on similar flights to Sollas, Campbeltown and Benbecula.

On 12th May David Barclay took the Heron for beach landings at Sollas and Harris to give route experience to Captain Paddy Calderwood for future ambulance flights. On 28th May an era ended with the last Rapide flight, an ambulance run to Campbeltown. On 27th October the Isle of Coll was surveyed and an ambulance flight followed on 4th December. However on another familiarisation flight, on 20th February 1957, G-ANXA was damaged on the island. In reporting the incident the press described what had occurred, 'The pilot, Captain P Calderwood, had to correct for a considerable amount of drift while making an approach on one of the island's two emergency landing strips. When the aircraft touched down its nose wheel collapsed. The two starboard engines were also damaged. None of the crew of three was injured.'

Flights to less regular landing grounds such as Coll, Oronsay and Harris seem to have ceased around this time. Some other airfields, particularly those on the northern isles of Orkney appear only ever to have featured for route training and were not used by BEA in the 1950s for regular ambulance cases.

Two births occurred on the Heron in 1957. One of these was on an aircraft diverted from its scheduled run to uplift an expectant mother from Benbecula. The second, on 18th July, was from the beach landing strip at Sollas on North Uist. Baby Alexander MacPherson was born upon touch-down at Renfrew.

Renfrew Airport transferred its scheduled services to the new civil airport at Abbotsinch in 1966 and there is now little to mark the site of Glasgow's former airport. But nestling in a housing estate where the street names nostalgically recall the turbo-prop airliners of the 1950s and 1960s, stands a simple cairn unveiled that year by the late Captain David Barclay MBE MStJ.

The cairn contains stones gathered from many of the Scottish islands and is dedicated to all those who served with the Scottish Air Ambulance Service from Renfrew Airport. On two sides of the cairn silhouettes of the de Havilland Rapide, designed by Avril Gibb of Skelmorlie, capture the flavour of early air ambulance flights.

But more specifically, the cairn commemorates a particular ambulance team which set out from Renfrew following a call from Islay on the night of 28th September 1957. That flight ended in tragedy when BEA's Heron G-AOFY *Sir Charles Bell* came down on approach to Islay's Glenegedale Airport in appalling weather conditions. On board were Captain Paddy Calderwood, Radio Officer Hugh McGinlay and Sister Jean Kennedy. None of them survived.

When word of the missing aircraft reached Glasgow's Southern General Hospital, Matron Isobel Wares took the call. The time was 1.00am.

'It was the most terrible night I ever remember. By the time I had dressed, they rang again to say the plane was lost with everyone on board. They wanted another nurse to fly out in a second ambulance.'

'How could I possibly ask anyone after what had happened? I wanted to go myself but the medical superintendent told me I was needed in the hospital to answer inquiries. He was right. The phone never stopped ringing for twenty-four hours. Every available nurse volunteered. I chose Sister Isobel Thompson, a junior night sister.'

By the time Sister Thompson arrived at the airport, the storm was so violent it was impossible for the aircraft even to take-off. Three hours later, BEA's Flight Manager, Captain Eric Starling, finally managed to get the second Heron airborne and the small aircraft struggled over to Islay. But as they returned to the mainland Sister Thompson came to realise that everyone's efforts had been in vain. The patient, Mrs Margaret McClugash, seriously ill with diabetes, died ten minutes before the plane touched down on the runway at Renfrew. It was the most disastrous night in the history of the air ambulance.

Captain Kenneth McLean, who had been posted to Renfrew earlier that year, joined Eric Starling on the flightdeck of the follow-up aircraft. 'I was living locally in digs with a Mrs Mason in a neat bungalow near the "back gate" of Renfrew Airport. She wakened me in the small hours one morning, saying that there was a phone call from the Air Ambulance for me to report to the airport. When I arrived, Captain Starling was already there. He imparted the news that a previous ambulance flight during the night had crashed on the way in to land at Islay and that the aircraft had been destroyed with all on board killed.'

'I went out with Captain Starling, picked up the patient and returned to Renfrew. We parked away from the terminal, as usual, and were hustled away in a car to avoid the Press who had got wind of the night's events by then. Some time previously Paddy Calderwood had been on the TV programme 'What's My Line?', and had done his bit of mime to denote tuning-in one of the radio navigation sets on the cockpit roof panel. I don't think any of the TV panel sussed out what his line was. I seem to recall that he had young twin daughters and had brought them in to Renfrew one day.'

The traumatic events of the night, recalls Eric Starling, resulted in an immediate change of policy. 'It tended to be at a crew's discretion as to whether they took to the air and this often meant ambulances setting off in conditions that were keeping all other aircraft grounded. But following the Islay crash, ambulance pilots would be required strictly to observe weather minima.'

Captain Geoff Northmore recalls one of the changes that resulted. 'A second pilot was carried after this time, replacing the role of the radio officer. I had to take my turn as First Officer-cum-Safety Pilot a couple of times each month. The Heron was then classified as a single pilot aircraft so all my type-flying is logged as "passenger". This did not prevent First Officers from physically handling the aircraft as we sat in the right hand cockpit seat where a control column and rudder pedals were fitted. In addition, by then, an airspeed indicator and altimeter were fitted on the starboard coaming for the First Officer's use and comfort in bad weather. No other instruments were fitted on the starboard side.'

Both BEA and later Loganair paid tribute to Jean Kennedy, a native of the Isle of Coll, by naming aircraft in her honour. At the Southern General Hospital, the management decided to award the 'Jean Kennedy Memorial Gold Medal' to the Best Nurse in 3rd Year Training. The first winner of the medal, in 1958, was Christina Ann MacRitchie from Barvas on the Isle of Lewis. 'It was with surprise and humility that I was deemed or chosen to be the first recipient of the medal. I was in bed with 'flu on the night of the crash on Islay and the memory of it is still vivid as Jean Kennedy was someone that we students always looked up to.'

At this time the practice of presenting 'wings' to nurses serving on the air ambulance began. One of the recipients at the first presentation was Ellen Hutchison. Matron at the Southern General, Isobel Wares, wrote to Nurse Hutchison on 18th November 1958 announcing the new award, 'Scottish Oils and Shell-Mex Ltd have presented us with a number of Silver Wings Badges to be presented to nurses who do a certain number of flights in the Air Ambulance Service. It was decided that the count should be taken from 1st May 1956, and that seven flights should have been completed to qualify for the badge. The presentation will take place on Friday 28th November 1958 at the end of the Prize-Giving ceremony. You have qualified for this badge and I should be very pleased if you were able to attend to receive your award.'

The requirement for the Silver Wings was later changed to ten ambulance flights but the tradition of presenting the award continued for the next thirty years during which the Southern General would continue to provide nurses for the service. Nurses from hospitals such as the Gilbert Bain Hospital in Lerwick and the Balfour Hospital in Kirkwall were also accorded the award, the only non-nursing college decoration permitted on a nurse's uniform.

In 1960 BEA reported that, in the previous year, refresher courses for nurses had been conducted in aviation medicine, emergency procedures, and survival training. The programme included familiarisation visits to the aircraft at Renfrew Airport. A total of 75 nurses from the Southern General had completed the courses.

The only material recognition that nurses could expect for accompanying air ambulance cases was an honorarium of One Guinea for each flight. In later years this became Two Pounds. Obviously nurses did not volunteer for ambulance flights for the financial reward. Comforting patients from remote parts of the country was their main concern — although the thrill of the journey by air may have been a welcome bonus.

Not infrequently other BEA aircraft had to be pressed into service for ambulance duties because the regular ambulance aircraft was already out on a call or was in the engineering bay. Dakotas (which BEA called the Pionair class) sometimes substituted for the Rapide; and Heralds or Viscounts upon occasion performed the tasks of the Heron.

Dakota Captain George Stone flew out of Renfrew in 1954/55. 'Eric Starling, BEA's Flight Manager, was always telling us how flying around the islands was a special kind of flying, quite different from what we were used to on the trunk routes, and how certain tricks could be helpful. On one occasion he told us that, if the wind was too strong, we could stop the Dakota at the end of the runway and the passengers would be brought out to the plane. And if it was really strong we could leave the flaps down and let the wind blow the aircraft back along the runway until it was opposite the terminal. I thought I'd never heard so much old bull — until I had to land at Stornoway in 70-80 knots, almost take-off speed. I decided to try letting the aircraft blow back along the runway, still very sceptical, but sure enough, it really worked.'

'During the period when the Herons were being taken on to replace the Rapides, Dakotas were used for some ambulance flights. On 13th January 1955 I flew one of these to Benbecula in a snow storm. The seriously ill patient was already at the airport as we circled overhead, awaiting a break in the blizzard. As we landed, the Pionair slithered across a four-inch covering of snow with the four-man fire crew standing by. It was not a normal landing.'

The patient, Mary MacEachan, had already endured an horrific journey to reach Benbecula Airport. For ambulance driver Mona McLennan this began with the 16-mile drive from Lochboisdale to Miss MacEachan's croft at Ardivachar through drifting snow. The patient then had to be carried by stretcher for more than half-a-mile from her isolated croft to the road. It was a further 14 miles to the airport.

Upon arrival at Renfrew Airport, 55 minutes after take-off from Benbecula, Nurse Elizabeth McLeod transferred her patient over to the road ambulance which rushed to Glasgow's Western Infirmary with a priest also in attendance. Meanwhile, back on Benbecula, the road ambulance there had to return to Lochboisdale. Dr G McKinnon was on board the ambulance, 'It was a nightmare journey back. You could not see where the road ended and the ditch began. There were drifts of four feet. Windscreen wipers were useless as the snow drove at you from all sides.'

Captain Jim McDonald had to use the 70-passenger Vickers Viscount to collect an expectant mother from Campbeltown. 'We were on finals to RAF Machrihanish in foul weather when Air Traffic Control came on to say that the Commanding Officer did not recommend a landing in these conditions. It was for our crews to make their own decisions on these matters and we touched down, coming to a halt half way up the runway. The road ambulance came out to us, stopped, . . . and then, nothing. We went to investigate to learn that the mother had been giving birth inside the ambulance. We returned to Glasgow without having collected our patient.'

Sister Jean Stalker recalls an air ambulance flight which had to come to the rescue of the regular scheduled service. 'We had flown a patient home from Edinburgh to Stornoway. On the return flight to Glasgow, the pilot was told to change course for Tiree. The plane booked for the regular afternoon passenger service was out of action and the ambulance plane had to take its place.'

'We picked up some passengers at Tiree and came down for more at Islay. A young airline official wanted a lift to Glasgow where he had a date with a girl friend. Unfortunately, all the seats were filled.'

'But he was very desperate to go, so the pilot asked me, "Would you mind if we carried him as a patient?"'

'It seemed a very pleasant idea so we got him on to the stretcher and strapped him down. All the way to Glasgow, the passengers kept looking at him and whispering, "The poor man".'

A similar event occurred in July 1954. Coll Macdonald had been a Traffic Clerk at Benbecula from 1950 until 1953, when he was transferred to Manchester. He then had to make an urgent visit back home because of the sudden death of his mother.

'This news reached me in the evening and I set off by train to Glasgow. My colleagues at Ringway contacted Renfrew with a request to try and get me on the flight to Benbecula the following morning. This was not to be as the aircraft was full. However I was told to hang around in case there might be a call for an ambulance. I did not have to wait for very long.'

'The destination was Stornoway and we set off with Bob Payne (ex Fleet Air Arm) in command. I was to catch the southbound service from Stornoway to Benbecula in the afternoon. But it was not quite as simple as that. Our aircraft developed a snag and we had to land at Tiree. The outcome was that we had to wait for the inbound service from Barra, switch aircraft and be on our way. Our original aircraft was obviously deemed fit to return to Renfrew.'

'While we were at Tiree I mentioned casually to Bob that I would be spending the night in Stornoway as we would arrive there too late to make my connection. I don't think he made any comment. Shortly after take-off from Tiree he told me to be ready to jump out as soon as he came to a halt on the runway at Benbecula. I am sure the wheels did not quite stop on that runway. And so it was that an ambulance aircraft made an unscheduled, unrecorded landing/touch-and-go at Benbecula!'

The nationalised airlines, BEA and BOAC, were frequently accused of not being business-orientated. Nonetheless the costs of running the air ambulance service, which were passed on to the Scottish Home and Health Department, had to be agreed by both parties as fair. Ronald Philpot, a Cost Accountant with BEA, had to make an annual visitation to the offices of the Department. 'It used to be my job to calculate the costs of operating the service, along with Robert McKean who was Manager Scotland for BEA. The costs used to increase year by year and we had to explain how we arrived at our figures and agree the cost of operations. The Department always eventually accepted our figures which were calculated with great care.'

Ambulance flights could be routine and even repetitive. But the best example of repetition was experienced when Captain Ken Browning flew to Benbecula on 6th November 1957 to bring in a young man with an eye injury caused by a firework. The nurse recognised him from a previous occasion. That time had also followed Guy Fawkes night when he had injured his other eye!

Islanders living off the Scottish mainland are extremely practical people, a characteristic that comes naturally to small communities balancing on a fragile economy. Ken Browning flew into Islay with the aid of goose-neck flares late one stormy winter's night. The weather was foul but the landing, to airlift an old lady in her eighties, was successful. She was put aboard the Heron and was accompanied by a young man introduced as her son.

They had not long taken off when the nurse came forward to the flight deck with the news that the old woman had died. On her heels was the young man saying, 'As ma mither's deid, can ye turn back as it'll be awfy expensive if we huv tae bring her back oorselves'. Ken Browning turned back into the storm towards Islay, hoping that the flares set out to mark the runway had not yet been extinguished.

On Saturday 30th May 1964 Jean Muir had been listening to her radio at her home in Orkney. News bulletins warned of a typhoid outbreak in Aberdeen, attributed to a batch of imported corned beef, and the rest of the nation was being advised to avoid visiting the city if at all possible. Over 200 cases of the epidemic had already been confirmed and the figure was rising daily. On the following day Jean was being whisked off from Kirkwall by air ambulance to give birth to her youngest child. Her destination — Aberdeen Maternity Hospital. But her visit took place without incident, unlike one which her air ambulance nurse had recently undertaken to Renfrew. That flight had resulted in the birth of a baby boy before reaching the hospital.

Geoff Northmore performed his first ambulance flight as First Officer to Captain Mike O'Brien on 3rd February 1960. 'It was to Campbeltown and I remember there was low cloud and snow. Mike gave me the leg back to Renfrew to give me my first night take-off and landing with the Heron. In bad weather the First Officer did the let down. He would fly the aircraft by leaning over to the left and using the captain's blind flying instruments. The captain would set the altimeter and reset the direction indicator for us. It worked very well but most First Officers disliked flying the Heron as we could not log the flying time and most of us needed hours in order to get higher pilot licences, so time in the Heron was wasted on us.'

It was on Herons that Captain Nick Wright received his first command with BEA at the end of 1970. 'We would often fly as low as 200 feet in the Heron when coming in from the islands, crossing the Crinan Canal and not encountering any obstruction until we reached Erskine Bridge. I continued flying with Herons until they were withdrawn and flew for a time on the Short SC7 Skyliners which replaced them.'

British Airways withdrew its two Herons, G-ANXA and G-ANXB, from service in 1973. Their ambulance role was then performed by Loganair with Britten-Norman Islanders. The scheduled service from Glasgow to Tiree and Barra, on which the Herons had also been used, was then operated by two Short Skyliner aircraft until 1975 when this service was also transferred to Loganair. An occasional ambulance flight was undertaken by British Airways with the Skyliner during the period of transition when the service was being transferred to Loganair, but these were small in number.

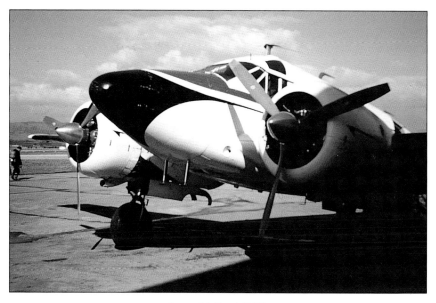

Loganair's Beech E18S
which performed some of the longer distance ambulance flights in the 1970s.
(Photo by Captain Ken Foster)
First production Britten-Norman Islander G-ATWU
which was to pioneer Loganair's air ambulance role.
(Photo courtesy of Tony Naylor)

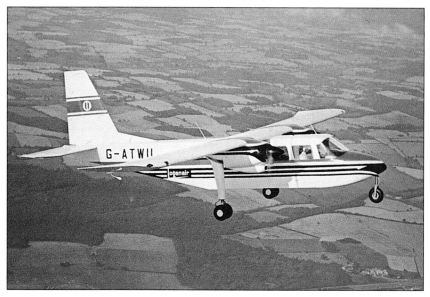

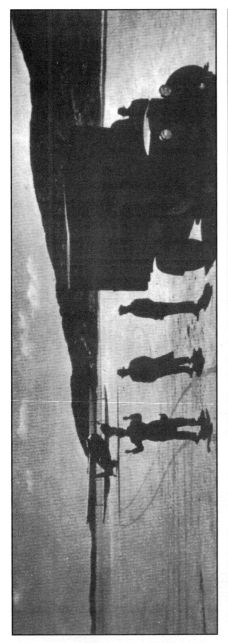
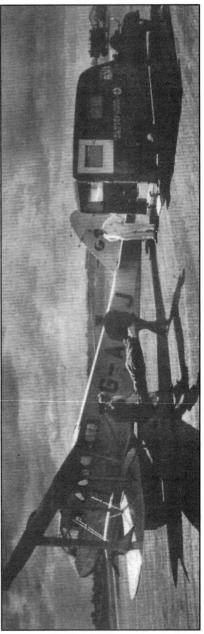

BEA Rapide taxies in at Barra. The truck serves as an improvised ambulance. *(Top)*
The patient is transferred to one of more conventional appearance at Renfrew. *(Bottom)*
(Photos Picture Post magazine courtesy of Mrs Wendy Johnson)

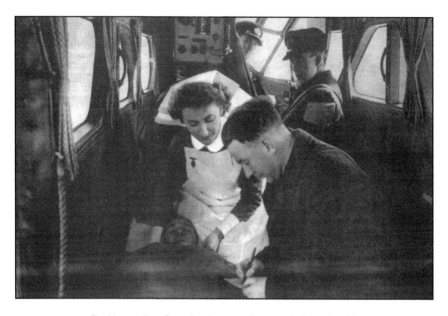

Final instructions from the doctor to the nurse before take-off
while Captain Bill Johnson awaits the O.K.
(Photo Picture Post Magazine courtesy of Mrs Wendy Johnson)

Captain Don Hoare and Radio Officer MacKenzie receive a Met. briefing at Renfrew.
(Photo BEA courtesy of Tony Naylor)

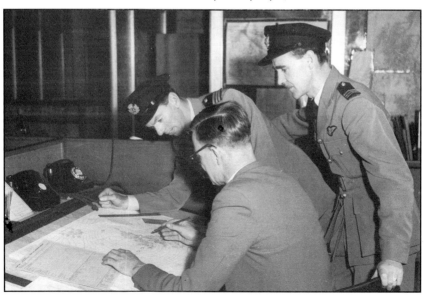

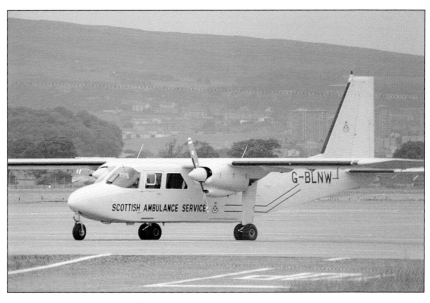

Loganair Islander in the colours of the Scottish Air Ambulance Service at Glasgow in 1994.
(Photo by the author)

Bond Aviation's Beechcraft Super King Air embarks a patient at Glasgow Airport in 1993.
(Photo by the author)

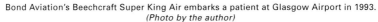

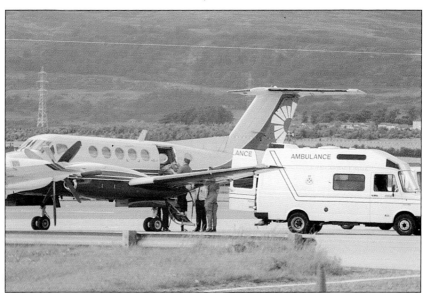

G-ANXA was leased to Sierra Leone Airways until 1974 when it was sold to Norwich-based oil support operator, Peters Aviation. In 1977 it passed on to Air North in New Zealand where it flew for a further two years. In 1981, while in storage there, it was set alight by vandals and destroyed.

G-ANXB was also sold to Peters Aviation and subsequently passed to other owners. It was withdrawn from service in 1979 and in 1981 was donated to the Newark Air Museum in Nottinghamshire where it remains on display, symbol of a past era.

The Scottish Office acknowledged the role played by BEA in a letter from the Secretary of State for Scotland, Gordon Campbell: 'There are many patients in the remoter areas of Scotland who have cause to be grateful to the aircrews in particular for their devotion to the service and their determination to get through to aid those in need of urgent treatment in hospital. But all the other members of the staff played their essential part also and deserve their share of our gratitude.'

To mark the role played by the nursing staff at Glasgow's Southern General Hospital, BEA's Robert McKean presented a model of the venerable Heron to Matron Isobel Wares. Miss Wares had co-ordinated the air ambulance nurses from the hospital for the last seventeen years.

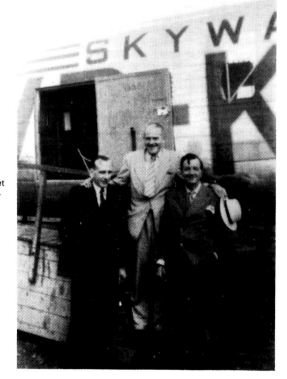

Deprived of their airline after nationalisation, former Scottish Airways directors Bill Cummings (Company Secretary), George Nicholson and Edmund Fresson meet up 'somewhere in Africa', in 1948. *(Photo courtesy of Sheila Harper)*

Islands and Islanders

The Air Ambulance and Loganair

THE PRE-WAR independent airlines had undertaken air ambulance flights to virtually any island which had need of this new aerial lifeline. All that was required was enough cleared ground on which to land the simple but versatile aircraft of the era. Following nationalisation, the service operated by BEA tended to be limited to the established airfields which it also served with regular scheduled flights.

But twenty years later Loganair, established in 1962 as an air taxi company, joined BEA in providing air ambulance cover, extending the service to islands where the larger airline's Herons were unable to operate.

Loganair's very first air ambulance flight was undertaken by Piper Aztec PA23-250C, G-ASYB, on 16th June 1967, when Captain Ken Foster uplifted a patient to Glasgow from the grass airstrip on the Isle of Oronsay. Ken Foster recalls the constraints encountered on that first flight because of the size of the aircraft, 'The launch of our air ambulance role was intended to coincide with the delivery of our first Britten-Norman Islander. However this was delayed due to the crash in the Netherlands of Britten-Norman's prototype of the aircraft. The Aztec offered very limited space and we had to install removable hinge pins in the door so that it could easily be taken off. The co-pilot's seat and centre seat were also removed to make room for the stretcher which had to be eased over the engine nacelle in order to load the patient on board at Oronsay.'

The arrival of the Britten-Norman BN2 Islander aircraft during the following month made Loganair a serious player in the arena of air ambulance operations. Loganair had worked closely with Britten-Norman Ltd in developing the Islander aircraft and took delivery of the first production model, G-ATWU, in July 1967. The STOL capabilities of this rugged aircraft made air ambulance flights to the most basic of airstrips possible.

From 1967 Loganair operated daylight air ambulance flights to the islands of Coll, Colonsay, Jura, and Mull. (Jack Armour of Tobermory, suffering from peritonitis, was the first patient to be uplifted from Mull when he was flown to Oban in the Piper Aztec on 1st August 1969.) The beach landing sites at Northton, Harris, and Sollas, North Uist, and the newly built airstrip at Plockton, Wester Ross, were also accessible by Loganair's Islander. While most would bring patients to Glasgow, some of Loganair's flights from the Inner Hebrides operated to North Connel airfield to deliver patients to the West Highland Hospital in Oban.

Ken Foster, Loganair's Operations Director, was keen to take the air ambulance service to areas which had not previously enjoyed access to it because of the limitations of local landing sites. In the south-west, airfields at Wigtown, Dumfries, Castle Kennedy, and West Freugh were surveyed and doctors were notified that the air ambulance could be made available to them. But old habits die hard and occasions arose when a seriously ill or injured patient was transported on a four-hour road journey from Dumfries-shire or Galloway when the Islander could have moved the patient with less discomfort and taken only thirty minutes.

Doctors on Skye also were slow to take up the facility offered by the air ambulance despite their having been less reticent in doing so when aircraft could land on the island during the 1930s. Indeed the arrival of a modern airfield on Skye was delayed when local officials insisted on it being sited near Portree although the town offered no suitable landing site while Broadford did. The airfield was to have been built under the OPMAC (Operation Military Aid to the Community) scheme with soldiers from engineer regiments doing the construction as part of annual exercises and the local council providing the materials.

While the soldiers waited on Skye for a decision on an airfield site, officials from Plockton needed no prompting. They offered a suitable landing area in Wester Ross where construction could begin immediately. The army moved their equipment across the water, and Skye had to await a new opportunity. Skye airfield was eventually built at Broadford and opened in 1972. By March 1973 the air ambulance had still not been called out to Skye yet some serious cases had been conveyed to Inverness by road.

Other areas were joining a waiting list for OPMAC-constructed airports and those whose aspirations remained unfulfilled when the scheme closed included Arran, Rothesay, Gigha, Daliburgh (South Uist), Durness, Morvern (Argyll), Canna, and Muck. The army engineers arrived on Arran in readiness to build an airstrip at Shiskine when a disagreement arose between the landowner and the local authority over the terms of the lease. It was not resolved, the engineers left the island, and a quarter of a century later Arran is still without an airfield.

A doctor on Harris immediately recognised the benefits offered by Loganair's Islander aircraft and periodically patients were uplifted from the beach at Northton. Pilots had to land once-annually on such airfields to qualify for a current operating permit; so a small pool of pilots would be established by a currently authorised pilot taking a co-pilot on such call-outs so that he too would be familiar with the airfield for the immediate future. In 1976 the first landing on Berneray in thirty years was undertaken by Ken Foster to test the cockle strand adjacent to Borve Machair for possible air ambulance use.

From the beginning, Loganair observed a policy of always trying to respond to a call. If the destination airport was closed because of the weather an aircraft would still take-off because conditions might improve during the flight, and if they did not, a landing would be made at the nearest alternative field until the weather cleared. If there was a night call to a strip without lights, pilots would take-off in darkness, having calculated the time of first light at the other end, so as to be able to uplift the patient as promptly as possible. Instances of defeat by the weather were very rare indeed.

At Campbeltown, if high winds were sweeping across the long operational runway and inhibiting a normal landing, the versatile Islander could land on a cross-taxiway. Ken Foster recalls a landing on Coll in winds of 55 knots, 'I was doubtful about landing at the regular airfield but saw possibilities of using a former landing site below Ben Feall. I advised the people on Coll where to expect me, to which our man remarked "It's a long time since we've come in there!" When I got down I had to "fly" the plane on the ground because of the wind. A tractor was placed at the nose of the aircraft to break the windflow and to stop the aircraft door being blown off while the patient was loaded. When we were loaded up, the tractor was pulled back and the aircraft did a vertical take-off.'

Loganair established a base at Kirkwall in 1967 where the Islander aircraft inaugurated Orkney inter-island scheduled services on similar principles to those previously established by Edmund Fresson and his Highland Airways during the 1930s, but abandoned by the new British European Airways Corporation when it was established in 1947. Twenty years absence of air ambulance cover ensured that the arrival of Loganair was greeted enthusiastically. Dr Derek Johnstone of Balfour Hospital in Kirkwall summed up the situation very well in a 1972 lecture about the benefits of the air ambulance, 'Before that patients travelled by sea. If they were not ill by the time they started the journey they were damned ill by the time they arrived.'

Orkney County Council set about creating airfields on its northern islands so that a comprehensive network was quickly established, providing landing sites on Eday, North Ronaldsay, Papa Westray, Sanday, Stronsay, and Westray. The council opened an airfield on the southern island of Hoy in 1972, while at various times other airstrips were established in conjunction with private owners on Egilsay, Flotta, Rousay, Shapinsay, and Wyre. Use of the Rousay strip was discontinued by Loganair after an Islander ended up in a ditch with a bent nose wheel after landing in wet conditions.

Captain Jim Lee, a colourful character who sported a bushy beard, was Loganair's first Orkney-based pilot. Jim Lee flew many early ambulance flights from the islands of Orkney. He later became a medical practitioner and, some years after, a Loganair pilot who landed on Tiree to uplift a patient found that the doctor who had placed the call was Dr Lee working on the island in the capacity of locum.

Jim Lee was succeeded in Orkney by Andy Alsop who was to become one of the aviation legends of the islands. Customarily, Loganair captains, as they gained greater seniority, were expected to relocate from such stations after a period so that they might move on to larger aircraft. But Andy Alsop discovered an affinity with Orkney that he was reluctant to lose and he remained there for many years. When the time to move could be postponed no longer, he found that flying around the Falklands and Antarctica was more to his liking than the busy skies of Glasgow or Aberdeen. In the 1990s he is therefore to be found flying in the South Atlantic during the Antipodean summer while he still maintains a home in Orkney.

Excerpts from some of the early air ambulance cases from the islands of Orkney include: 'Injured youth collided on his motor-cycle with a cow on Sanday (the cow was killed)', 'Badly scalded baby flown from North Ronaldsay to hospital in Aberdeen', 'Stronsay's oldest resident, aged 97, flown to Kirkwall after sustaining a fractured skull (declining a stretcher and boarding the aircraft herself)'. It is worth pondering what options would have been available to these patients had there been no air ambulance.

The airstrip constructed on the island of Hoy was soon being used for ambulance flights as well as scheduled services. The new strip was first put to use in this role in May 1973 when Andy Alsop uplifted the mate of the salvage vessel *Dispenser*. Before the opening of the airstrip, it would have been necessary to convey the sick man to the Orkney mainland in the Longhope lifeboat.

A rough voyage in a lifeboat was the daunting prospect in store for Lesley and Michael Scott, aged five and two, who were suspected of swallowing camphor balls while playing at their North Ronaldsay home. The island was blanketed in fog making an air landing impossible and the Kirkwall lifeboat set out on the forty-mile trip to North Ronaldsay. Captain Jamie Bayley decided to attempt a flight when the fog lifted slightly and he reached North Ronaldsay just as the lifeboat was arriving. Jamie flew the children, accompanied by their father, directly to Aberdeen where they recovered in the Sick Children's Hospital.

Shapinsay did not present such problems because of its proximity to Kirkwall. The flying time to Kirkwall Airport was only two and a half minutes, but patients could be conveyed to hospital just as speedily by sea. The air ambulance only became first choice when the sea conditions were bad or when a patient had to be taken further afield. This was the case when Loganair's first evacuation from Shapinsay occurred in 1976 and Andy Alsop flew a woman patient direct to Aberdeen from the island's grass strip.

Loganair commemorated many new air services or events with the issue of special philatelic covers. Andy Alsop was particularly astute at identifying significant occasions, the most famous being the recording of the Westray-Papa Westray scheduled service in the *Guinness Book of Records* as the world's shortest scheduled flight. Ambulance flights were also acknowledged on philatelic envelopes which Andy always seemed to have bundled up in his flight bag for overprinting whenever a noteworthy event arose.

The island of Flotta was twice acknowledged in this way by ambulance flights. The first flight to the island was an ambulance operated by Islander G-AWNR on 28th May 1976 when Willie Barnett was flown to hospital in Kirkwall by Captain Alsop and Nurse Irene Skea. Then on 10th December of the same year the first night flight to Flotta was a visit by Islander G-AXKB making an ambulance call.

One event for which a first day cover was not issued, but which would have been worthy of such acknowledgement, was Loganair's first inflight birth. This happened on 2nd August 1973 at 2,000 feet above Kirkwall while Captain Jamie Bayley was flying Freida Devin from Stronsay to hospital in Aberdeen. The occasion was suitably marked when the baby girl, weighing in at 9lb 2oz, was named Katy Ferguson *Leynair* Devin to honour both Captain Bay*ley* and Loga*nair*.

Loganair's first international air ambulance flight took place from Orkney when Captain Peter Knudsen airlifted his 17-year-old countryman Odd Arne Lindgren to Bergen. Lindgren's leg had been severely crushed by a ship at Stromness harbour a week earlier and he had been taken to hospital in Kirkwall. Peter Knudsen was working alongside Alan Whitfield in Shetland at the time and he flew from Sumburgh to collect the young seaman.

During 1974 there was a long industrial dispute involving the fire services at Aberdeen's Dyce Airport. As a result, the airport was closed daily from 9.50pm until 7.00am. During the first few weeks of the strike the Civil Aviation Authority permitted Loganair to land air ambulance aircraft during these hours without fire cover. However this arrangement threatened to escalate the dispute. Several cases from the Northern Isles were affected. Orkney patients would be flown from the outer isles to Kirkwall where they would spend the night in the Balfour Hospital before continuing to Aberdeen next day. This arrangement was not suitable for one urgent case and Jamie Bayley flew his patient directly from Westray to Glasgow, arriving at 12.30am after a flight lasting two hours and forty minutes.

Shetland did not have the pre-war tradition of internal air services that Orkney had. Therefore to establish airfields around the islands of the Shetland group meant breaking totally fresh ground. The first strip to be opened was that at Unst which was completed by the Royal Engineers under the OPMAC scheme in 1968. However the local authorities in Shetland reflected a maritime tradition which was so strong that they did not embrace the development of inter-island air services with the same enthusiasm as did their counterparts in Orkney.

The response of local Shetland island communities, on the other hand, was very different and they strove eagerly to satisfy Loganair's requirements so that the airline could provide them with scheduled services and ambulance flights. Local communities made arrangements to make the most suitable fields available for landings and, once these had been surveyed, they turned out in force to remove walls and level ground to create an airstrip.

The first rough strips were completed in 1969 on Foula, Out Skerries, and Papa Stour. Additional airstrips were to follow on Fetlar, Whalsay (where the first ambulance flight took place in December 1972 to convey a two-year-old child to hospital in Lerwick) and Fair Isle. In 1976 the local authority completed a new landing strip at Tingwall on the outskirts of Lerwick.

The difference made by airstrips to outlying islands is ideally illustrated on Foula. 'I landed on Foula with the Christmas mail one year — in February. The island had been stormbound until then', recalls Ken Foster. 'There was no doctor on the island and the district nurse had to attend to any islanders in times of illness. With an ageing population, Foula was slowly dying, but within months of the airstrip being cut and access to swift evacuation to hospital by air in time of emergency being established, the island was recording the first increase in population in decades. I put this down directly to the new security and peace of mind that the air ambulance now provided.'

Driving force behind the creation of airmindedness in the outlying communities of Shetland was Captain Alan Whitfield. Soft-spoken and modest, Alan immersed himself fully in the Shetland community, which he remembers as being a very close one in the days before the first North Sea oil discoveries were making any impact on the islands. The flying appealed to him, 'Because you're not shut up in the sharp end of the aircraft on the Islander. You get to meet and to know the passengers.'

Assistance for the very first landing on Foula came from an unlikely source — Ken Gear, the island's ferryman. Alan was reluctant to cross to Foula by sea to survey a landing site in case he was stranded there by the island's unpredictable weather and he might be unable to return to the Shetland mainland in time to carry out his regular flying programme. Ken volunteered to lay out the makeshift 400-feet airfield, marking its 45-foot width with rocks which were then whitewashed.

The first landing was watched in awe by the islanders but Alan was delighted with it. 'It was a fairly simple landing. I could see the white stones clearly from well up. After taking a good look at the lie of things, I banked and headed in. The plane went down beautifully. The turf was quite firm, though it had been raining heavily for a few days, so I think it unlikely that we will ever get bogged down on the strip.' First medevac beneficiary of Foula's new airstrip was Leslie Bordman, a youngster on the island participating in an adventure holiday. His holiday had turned to misadventure when he sustained severe bleeding caused when he put his arm through a window.

With Alan's guidance and encouragement, the people of Papa Stour set to with a vengeance to level a landing site with picks and shovels. On Out Skerries the cost of laying an airstrip was calculated at £10,000. The island's twenty-five households immediately dug deep and produced £1,275 to set the project in motion.

Getting airstrips established was Alan's first mission on Shetland. But once they were up and running it took severe conditions indeed to prevent him coming to the aid of medical cases.

His determination was put fully to the test in March 1975 when two-year-old Annette Moncrieff was to be flown to Aberdeen with suspected paraquat poisoning. Alan had to abandon his vehicle on the way to Sumburgh Airport because the approaches were blocked by snowdrifts. The airport firemen, called out to cover the flight, also had to approach on foot. The aircraft was prepared for take-off but there was no sign of the young patient.

A police Landrover eventually found her father stranded near Robin's Brae. A snowplough had to be called to clear the way and it was in a Landrover of British Airways Helicopters that tiny Annette was driven to the awaiting Islander. Annette arrived at Aberdeen at 1.15am where she was soon reported to be out of danger.

The Glasgow-based Islander would often operate as far north as Orkney and Shetland. This was sometimes necessary as the Shetland crew might be about to find themselves 'out of hours' for the next day's scheduled services. In one strange sequence of events, the Shetland-based Islander flew to Orkney to fly a patient to Aberdeen as the Kirkwall-based aircraft was already en route to Aberdeen in response to an earlier call from Hoy. Needless to say, a call-out then came from Shetland, which had to be answered by an Islander from Glasgow, to evacuate a third case from the Northern Isles — to Aberdeen.

Between 1967 and 1973, BEA continued to be retained by the Scottish Home and Health Department to have an aircraft on 24-hour standby at Glasgow in readiness to depart to Campbeltown, Islay, Tiree, Barra, Benbecula, Stornoway, Wick, Kirkwall, or Sumburgh, their regular airfields for air ambulance call-outs. But from this period Ken Foster has memories of telephone messages during the night on several occasions to take a Loganair Islander out to one of the BEA fields. 'I would phone Gil Fraser, our Engineering Director, and the hospital to confirm that a nurse was on the way. Gil and I would then meet at the airport, push back the heavy hangar door and wheel the aircraft out by hand. This was completed within about thirty minutes of the call and the aircraft would usually be ready to go when the taxi carrying the nurse from the Southern General rolled up. We would also arrange a packed meal for the nurse who might have been on duty in the ward for eight hours and was now embarking on a night flight that might not return for another five.'

When BEA, now absorbed into British Airways, finally retired its de Havilland Herons in 1973, the Scottish Home and Health Department awarded the full air ambulance contract to Loganair. This took effect from 1st April and an Islander for ambulance duties was stationed at Glasgow, 24 hours per day, 365 days of the year. Two day-time crews for the service were on standby at Glasgow Airport, rostered from 0800 until 1500, and from 1500 until 2200. The night roster pilot, on duty between 2200 hours and 0800 hours, would normally cover from home, provided that the aircraft could be airborne within the hour.

A retainer was paid by the Department for the provision of one aircraft at Glasgow on round-the-clock availability while charter rates were paid for the use of service aircraft based in Orkney and Shetland, and this arrangement was extended to those at Inverness and Stornoway when required.

While BEA was sorry to lose the air ambulance contract which it had operated for a quarter of a century, there was goodwill all round for the successful transfer of this vital service. 'We wish Loganair well', said BEA Scottish Division Chairman, Robert McKean. 'They are not newcomers to the air ambulance service — for some years now they have been associated with us in this work. We will be pleased to offer them all the assistance we can in achieving a smooth handover. For this is not a proper subject for inter-airline rivalry. People's lives are at stake and there is no doubt that many hundreds of people in the remoter parts of Scotland owe their lives to the service.' Loganair showed its appreciation of that co-operation and support by naming one of its Islander aircraft after Robert McKean.

Loganair's Managing Director was obviously elated at the award of the full contract to what was still a small fledgling airline, 'We have arrived. And on 1st April when we take over the air ambulance work, we will have the final accolade of respectability', said Duncan McIntosh. 'We are very pleased and proud to have been chosen for this very important service and are very conscious of the traditions which BEA and their predecessors have built up. We will certainly do our best to maintain the standards set by them.'

As had occasionally been the case with BEA with their Herons, Loganair has from time to time deployed aircraft other than the Britten-Norman Islander for its ambulance duties. The Piper Aztec G-ASYB performed some of the earliest flights; but also used in an ambulance role occasionally was Loganair's Beech E18S, G-ASUG, until it was gifted into retirement at the Royal Scottish Museum. The Islander had been used to take transplant patients to Birmingham and Cambridge, but when Loganair acquired the Beech E18S to operate a scheduled service to Stavanger, it was also a much more suitable choice for these transplant ambulance flights or other long distance flights such as one in 1974 from Sumburgh to Newcastle to transfer a patient between hospitals.

From 1977 the DHC-6 Twin Otter would be used for ambulance duties when longer range flights were required. Again this would often happen when transplant patients were matched with donor organs and required quick transportation to hospitals in the south of England specialising in this type of surgery.

Captain David Marris, who flew several hundred air ambulance flights during his period with Loganair from 1977 until 1986, recalls two of these. 'In November 1985 I flew a

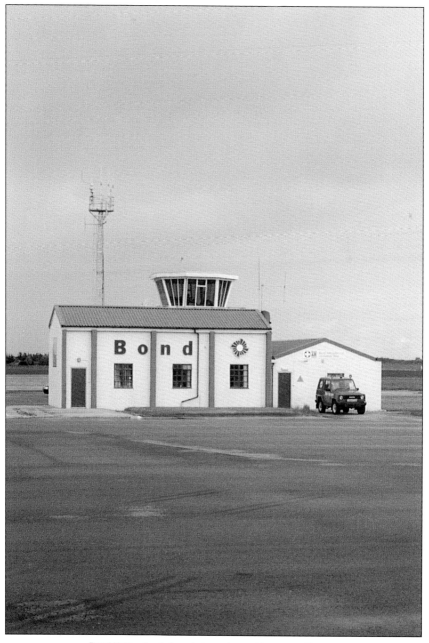

Bond Helicopters' air ambulance base at Inverness Airport.
(Photo by the author)

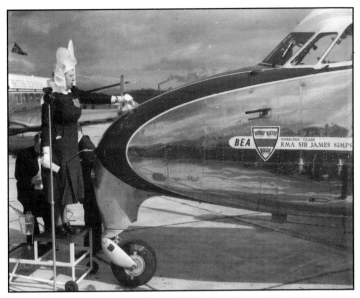

Matron Jean Jolly of Glasgow's Southern General Hospital
performs the naming ceremony of BEA's newly delivered De Havilland Herons in 1955.
(Photo BEA, courtesy of Tony Naylor)

Captain Ian Montgomery discusses his flight plan
with the nurse assigned to his next ambulance call-out.
(Photo BEA, courtesy of Captain Ian Montgomery)

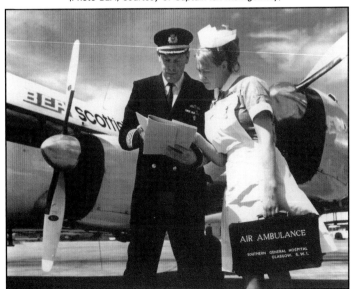

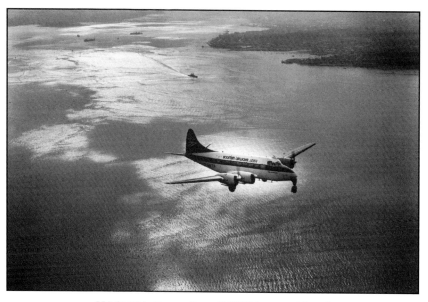

BEA Scottish Airways Heron G-ANXA homeward bound
over the Firth of Clyde.
(Photo BEA, courtesy of Tony Naylor)

'You don't expect me to lie down on that, do you?'
(Photo BEA, courtesy of Captain Ian Montgomery)

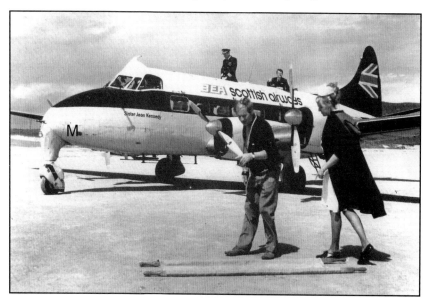

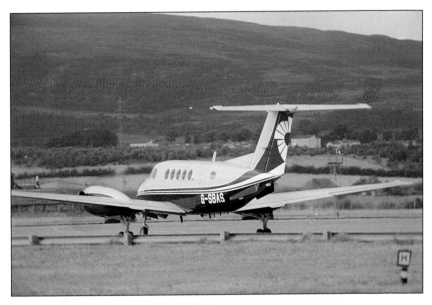

Bond's Beechcraft Super King Air taxies to the runway.
(Photo the author)

Dundee-based Bölkow BO 105D on the shores of a loch in 1989.
(Photo by Gerry Kelly)

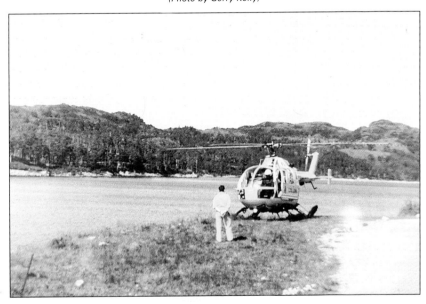

little boy, accompanied by his parents, to London Heathrow for a heart transplant. We left Glasgow at 2033hrs and returned at 0124hrs, having spent a total of four-and-a-quarter hours in the air. By way of contrast, I took a patient for a heart and kidney transplant to a small airfield at Alconbury, near Huntingdon, the following March, also in the larger DHC-6 Twin Otter. The Twin Otters had the seats removed nightly for mail flights and therefore the interiors could be adapted with equal ease to accommodate a stretcher.'

Captain Ben Bamber's experience of a Twin Otter ambulance was in very different circumstances. 'Three young people had been involved in an horrific car accident on Tiree. The seats were quickly removed from an Otter to permit the installation of three stretchers for a multiple evacuation.'

Because of demands on aircraft, other aircraft types, such as the Short SC7 Skyvan (1969-1973) and the Britten-Norman Mk III Trislander (1973-1982), would occasionally be pressed into air ambulance service. 'On one occasion in 1977 we had six aircraft airborne simultaneously in answer to ambulance calls taking them to points scattered from Campbeltown to Unst', recalls Ken Foster. 'The sudden demand was such that it created a shortage of the specially prepared bags of medical equipment which the Southern General Hospital always kept in readiness for the air ambulance nurses.'

History repeated itself in several respects in 1990 when Dr Robert Martin, then a junior doctor working in the surgical unit at the Southern General Hospital, was called to act as medical escort to a patient being transferred from Glasgow Royal Infirmary to Papworth Hospital for a heart transplant. As it happened, Dr Martin was working in the very wards and theatre where he first saw the light of day after his mother had been flown from Campbeltown in 1965 in labour as a medical emergency. 'Although ill from his cardiac problem, the patient was in no danger and so I sat in the co-pilot's seat of the Islander operated by Loganair for the flight. The pilot was from the Falkland Islands and had flown Islanders for years. He had a very ''colonial'' type of accent which was difficult to hear over the intercom. Nevertheless I enjoyed the trip and the constant chat heard over the radio which thankfully was medically uneventful.' The pilot with the colonial accent was Andy Alsop temporarily back at Loganair during a break from flying for the Royal Antarctic Survey interrupted by the southern winter.

While pilots make numerous uneventful ambulance flights, few of them do not have cases that are remembered vividly. The most poignant flight for David Marris took him to Wick to collect a badly burned father and son. 'The mother and a daughter had died in a house fire and the smell of charred flesh from the father and son was very noticeable. That one was very sad and definitely worthwhile.' David recalls flying another patient from Islay following a heart attack, only to lose him before he could be transferred from the aircraft to the road ambulance in Loganair's hangar at Glasgow Airport.

Kitty Macpherson was Loganair's first Station Manager at Barra, as she had previously been with BEA and British Airways until they relinquished the scheduled service from Glasgow in 1975. Kitty was well used to despatching her fellow islanders on the air ambulance in times of illness. She had been doing so for a long time, right back to 1936 when the planes of Northern & Scottish Airways were the ones that she was guiding on to the sands of Tràigh Mhòr. She recalled, 'All the people on Barra used to collect money at concerts and cèilidhs to put into a communal fund for ambulance flights when they were necessary.' In 1980 Kitty suffered a stroke and found herself on board Loganair's Islander, bound for Glasgow's Southern General Hospital. Philosophically she commented, 'Never did I think I would be one of the lucky ones to have first-hand experience of the service.'

Twin Otter pilot Jack Long undertook an ambulance flight on a singular occasion which made the memory of it and its particular circumstances all the more vivid. 'It was on New Year's Eve, 31st December 1979. At 1400 hrs I was scrambled in Twin Otter G-BELS, taking off from Aberdeen at 1424 and landing forty minutes later at Inverness. We did not get away until fifty-nine minutes later at 1523 as we had to detach some rear seats to load an incubator with a new baby, accompanied by mother and doctor. We only took thirty minutes back to Aberdeen and parked nose in at the "new" terminal paralleling 24 Runway to shield the passengers and ambulance from a strong north-westerly.'

'I rang the hospital later to hear the worst possible news. The poor little mite had not made it through the night. This caused New Year's Day to be a bit more of a blur than usual as it reminded me too much of losing a three-year-old son in 1968 and a still-born baby girl two-and-a-half years later. Knowing how this affected my wife and our daughter, my heart went out to that mother and the despair the New Year must have brought.'

Some patients are reluctant to board a plane despite, or maybe because of, their need for urgent medical attention. Dave Dyer recalls one unwilling passenger. 'We had landed on one of the smaller Hebridean islands. Gisela Thürauf was the nurse and, as was her habit when we had to await the arrival of the patient, she wandered off for a stroll round the airfield examining the local flora. The doctor then arrived with his charge, a frail lady in her eighties. But she was strenuously resisting all attempts to get her to the aircraft. The doctor explained that this was because of the effect of the drugs that he had had to administer and he decided that another injection would calm her down for the flight. As soon as he had given this additional injection, the frail octogenarian shot off down the airfield with the rest of us trailing in pursuit. Nurse Thürauf saw what was happening and was able to intercept her, but only with a rugby tackle. The old lady came quietly after that.'

For pilots to don robe and mask if they were flying an infectious case was not unknown. The flightdeck of the Islander is not separated from the cabin as was the case with the Heron. Patient contact with the pilot could also be a hazard with psychiatric cases. One such patient made a grab at a pilot's neck from behind, causing a few moments of alarm. Captains wore clip-on detachable neckties following that incident.

The early respect which Loganair gained for its development of the air ambulance service was acknowledged in the award of three Queen's Commendations for Valuable Service in the Air. Captain Ken Foster gained his for the identification and advancing of new landing sites throughout Scotland while Captain Alan Whitfield's award was in appreciation of the very specialist development work that he had carried out in Shetland. The third award went to Nurse Gisela Thürauf, a charismatic personality who flew hundreds of flights on the Islanders and the Herons that preceded them. Gisela lived for the air ambulance and to mark her achievement of 500 flights she was awarded a unique set of gold wings by Duncan McIntosh. When she retired from nursing she had flown more than 900 air ambulance missions.

Dr Bill Clegg of Tobermory on the Isle of Mull was voicing sentiments that could be echoed by others throughout Scotland when he wrote to Duncan McIntosh in 1974. 'Once again I must write to thank you on behalf of the people of the island for the splendid service provided on Sunday morning. In extremely difficult conditions a spendidly smooth operation was carried out thereby enabling a critically ill patient to get to Glasgow and thus giving him his only chance of recovery. Would you please pass on to the Captain of the aircraft my sincere thanks for his excellent performance under what I am sure were extremely trying conditions.'

In April 1993, Loganair's air ambulance role was temporarily restricted to operations from its Orkney and Shetland bases, following the introduction of the Bölkow BO 105D helicopters at Prestwick and Inverness. But a Glasgow based Islander was re-introduced by popular demand of island doctors in November 1993, now painted in the distinctive colours of the Scottish Ambulance Service, equipped with the latest life-saving apparatus and with SAS paramedics accompanying each flight.

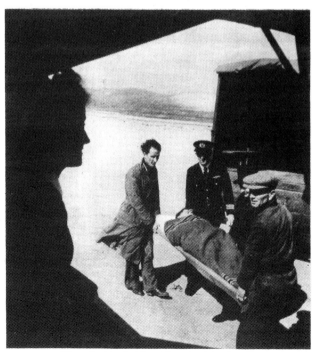

The patient is stretchered from truck to aircraft.
(Photo Picture Post magazine courtesy of Mrs Wendy Johnson)

The Helicopter Ambulance

*I*N APRIL 1993 much publicity was given to the launch of a 'new' air ambulance service, with strong emphasis on helicopters, to be operated by Aberdeen-based Bond Helicopters Ltd, following the success of its application by tender. Bond was established in 1972 as North Scottish Helicopters and had offshore SAR experience dating from 1983 resulting from contracts for British Petroleum in the Forties Field and Elf Petroleum in the Frigg Field.

Bond's air ambulance experience in Scotland had begun with an experimental service based at Dundee from 4th April 1989 on a six-month trial basis. The project, costing £190,000, of which British Telecom provided £110,000 in a sponsorship deal, put the specially equipped Bölkow BO 105D of Bond Helicopters within immediate range of Tayside, Fife, and Lothian but with the ability to operate to any part of Scotland, should the need arise. The Tayside operation in turn was able to benefit from the experience of the Cornish Air Ambulance which began in 1987 and is also operated by Bond. Both operations were branded *First Air*.

Yet the idea went back much further than that. In December 1952 the Northern Regional Hospital Board announced that it was to arrange a survey of possible landing places in the Highlands and Islands at which a helicopter could land with a view to introduction within five years.

And in 1971, Tony Naylor, Operations Manager of BEA's Scottish Airways Division, was interested in exploring the latest helicopters with a view to employing them on the Scottish Air Ambulance Service. 'The ability of the helicopter to transfer a patient directly from the scene of an accident to the grounds of the hospital would have reduced trauma quite considerably', recalls Naylor. 'I created the cautious interest of the Scottish Home and Health Department and I arranged a visit of their representatives to Munich in 1972. The machine they inspected there was the Bölkow BO 105.'

No immediate conclusion was reached and the following year the air ambulance contract passed to Loganair to be operated by its Britten-Norman Islander aircraft. Yet Tony Naylor's assessment remained just as relevant 17 years later.

As a consequence of the Scottish Ambulance Service link-up with Bond Helicopters, the place of the traditional volunteer air ambulance nurse was taken over by paramedics trained to give life-support in emergencies. The helicopter displayed its versatility by operating in co-ordination with road ambulances, sometimes playing a dual role with its wheeled counterpart in taking a patient from the scene of an accident to hospital, or in transporting between hospitals urgent items such as donor organs for transplant.

John Wilby was Director of the Scottish Ambulance Service at this time and his enthusiasm for the helicopter enabled the Dundee trial to become a reality. Additional help with the practical problems of an innovation of this nature came from Paul Westaway of the Cornish Air Ambulance.

Joining Captain Phil Green for the very first helicopter air ambulance calls from Dundee were paramedics Gerry Kelly and Ian Smith. The role of the paramedics is a demanding one and peak physical fitness is essential. The paramedics have at least two years' experience on road ambulances before taking to the air. Training includes an offshore survival course at the Robert Gordon Institute of Technology in Aberdeen, and Bond Helicopters' own air training course which covers air safety, navigation, and meteorology.

The very first mission was a simple transfer of a patient from Bridge of Earn Hospital to King's Cross Hospital, Dundee. But this was quickly followed by a flight that demonstrated the merits of the helicopter. At 1207 a call was received to take a man injured in an accident from Meikle to Dundee Royal Infirmary. The casualty arrived at the hospital at 1254.

Speed was paramount on 6th May 1989 when 21-month-old Amy Donaldson was savaged by a dog at Blairgowrie. The dog took off part of the toddler's nose. Amy's father fortunately picked up the piece of nose which was promptly packed in ice. Forty-five minutes later Amy was in Dundee Royal Infirmary where she was re-united with her nose. Paramedics Ian Golding and Gerry Kelly, along with pilot Phil Green. went to check on Amy's progress later that evening and found her making a rapid recovery.

Another early and grateful recipient of the service offered by the Dundee-based helicopter was Mrs Muriel Robertson. She had been at the wheel of her car at Kirriemuir when it was struck by an oncoming vehicle whose driver's attention had momentarily been distracted as he changed a tape casette. His lapse of concentration was nearly fatal for Muriel who feels she owes her life to the speedy arrival of the British Telecom-supported ambulance helicopter.

'The helicopter had been on its way to collect a patient from Brechin when the accident happened. The helicopter was re-directed mid-flight to Kirriemuir and rushed me off to Dundee Royal Infirmary. I was barely conscious of what was happening but I recall being aware of the "whirr" of the rotor blades. I would not have survived that crash had it not been for the helicopter.'

The helicopter experiment in Dundee was quickly voted a success but the renewal of sponsorship funding it presented a new challenge at the end of the six-month trial period and the conclusion of British Telecom's period of financial support. The Tayside Ambulance Service attracted some other sponsors to continue the helicopter operation for a few additional weeks. Companies were encouraged to sponsor the service for a week at a cost of £5,000. One company responding to this challenge was GB Papers Ltd of St Andrews — one of their employees had recently been killed in a road accident and this was a tangible way by which to remember him. The philanthropic input of Bond Helicopters in sustaining the service when funding became scarce was a gesture of its own faith in this type of operation which was soon emulated in the West Midlands of England, and in Devon.

However, on 1st February, Phil Green and his twin-engined Bölkow BO 105D moved to a new operational base at Inverness. This was to be for a one-month trial period but the relocation soon became permanent. The area being served now consisted of the Highlands and Islands, Aberdeenshire, and Tayside with patients being flown to Raigmore Hospital, Inverness, and occasionally to Belford Hospital, Fort William.

On 20th November 1991, Phil flew a motorist, whose car had struck a wall, from Nairn to Raigmore Hospital in Inverness. It was the 500th flight of the Bölkow BO 105D since its move to Inverness earlier in the year. Four more flights ferried patients to Raigmore Hospital that day, from Golspie, Helmsdale, Thurso, and Strathpeffer.

Dundee-based paramedics such as Ian Smith, Paul Gallen, Mike Knell, and John Lyall took turns to serve at Inverness for the first three months until paramedics from the Inverness area gained experience on helicopter operations. The first of these were Andy Fuller and David Haggerty.

Two months later another milestone was reached when baby Mark Waugh was born while his mother's helicopter journey from Kyle of Lochalsh to Inverness was still in progress.

Phil Green tells what happened, 'The baby's mother was in danger of going into labour two-and-a-half months early and her doctor wanted us to fly her to Raigmore where they could do something to help.'

'He assured us there was no chance of the child being born imminently but during the flight it became obvious that the baby had different ideas. I had to land the helicopter on the mountains alongside Loch Mullardoch approximately 25 miles west of Inverness.' Mark was delivered by air crew paramedics Kenny MacKenzie and David Haggerty. His birth was not straight forward and he had to be resuscitated throughout the rest of the journey, but thanks to the skill and speed of all concerned, Mark survived his unscheduled arrival into the world.

The wider application of helicopters was inaugurated in April 1993 following the announcement that the Scottish Ambulance Service had awarded a new contract worth £1.8 million annually. Dedicated Bölkow BO 105D helicopters operated by Bond Helicopters Ltd would fly from bases at Inverness and Prestwick while an Aérospatiale Dauphin SA 365C helicopter based at Plockton would be available on a non-dedicated basis. This would bring most parts of the Scottish mainland and the Western Isles within 30 minutes flying time of one of the three helicopter bases. At Aberdeen, Bond would also provide a fixed-wing Beechcraft King Air which would have a specific role for longer distance ambulance flights.

Loganair would continue to operate two Islanders in the Northern Isles where dedicated ambulance aircraft would be based at Kirkwall and Lerwick. After 26 years in this role, the now veteran Islander still remained the most suitable fixed-wing aircraft to operate in the rugged conditions often confronted in the air ambulance role.

── *Air Ambulance* ───────────────────────────────

The Scottish Ambulance Service would now control the whole operation by setting up an air desk at Aberdeen which became the doctor's first point of contact. The air desk could then provide a co-ordinated service, identifying the most suitable aircraft that should respond in each instance and also liaising with the Ministry of Defence or HM Coastguard when their help might be needed.

The new service was inaugurated with a special fly-past at Prestwick Airport, presided over by Lord Fraser of Carmyllie, Scottish Office Health Minister, and attended by such veterans of the service as Captain Eric Starling who had flown his first air ambulance flight in 1936, and Miss Margaret Boyd who flew as an air ambulance nurse between 1938 and 1942.

The helicopters brought a new versatility to the service. They could land almost anywhere, saving critical time when attending accidents in remote locations or even in urban areas where traffic congestion would impede road ambulances. Paramedics on board could provide immediate medical aid at the scene of an incident. The helicopter could then take patients directly to hospitals where simple helipads were designated in adjacent grounds or car parks.

Some regions of Scotland lacked airstrips and were faced with long road distances to the nearest hospital. Dumfries, Galloway, and the Borders, for example, could now benefit from a service from which they had previously been excluded. This was amply illustrated on 15th October 1993 when Barry Lockwood, an electricity worker, slipped as he unhooked a cable 80 feet up a disused pylon near Moffat and was injured as he fell against the framework. Three firemen and two paramedics scaled the pylon to reach the injured man who was then flown by air ambulance helicopter to the Intensive Care Unit at Dumfries Infirmary.

The Dauphin is a much larger machine than the Bölkow BO 105D and it is contracted to the Ministry of Defence for which it operates from its Plockton base. However it is put at the disposal of the Scottish Ambulance Service when required, subject to it being available. When such a need arises, a mobile ambulance unit kept in readiness at Plockton is installed in the Dauphin so that it is equipped to the same high standards as are to be found in the dedicated ambulance Bölkow BO 105D.

The pressurised Beechcraft King Air, provided by Bond under the new contract, operates from Aberdeen Airport and is employed on some of the longer distance ambulance flights where higher levels of speed and comfort might be of special importance. These might involve the transfer of organ transplant patients to hospitals in the south of England, or other hospital transfers to move patients to sources of specialist treatment or to closer proximity of their own homes. But the King Air is not just a ferry aircraft and is just as likely to be found evacuating a road accident victim from a Shetland airfield near the scene of the incident to hospital in Aberdeen.

Bond has two King Air aircraft and these are employed on a wide range of tasks. The arrangement with the Scottish Ambulance Service is that one of them can always be reserved by the SAS air desk and be fitted out for an air ambulance flight at five hours' notice. In reality Bond often succeeds in having one of these aircraft available within the hour if urgency demands an immediate response.

Loganair's pilots and ground staff had been extremely committed to the air ambulance service for many years and some staff undoubtedly took their diminished role badly. Some users of the service also found fault with the dedicated helicopters, particularly their inability to operate in darkness or in poor visibility, and the absence of space to accommodate an accompanying family member comfortably. The weather factor, or the lack of 24-hour helicopter cover, resulted in the Northern Isles-based Islanders making frequent visits to other parts of Scotland.

A further review therefore took place as 1993 progressed, and from 15th November, Loganair re-opened its air ambulance base at Glasgow Airport. Doctors and patients would therefore now have the benefit of both types of operation and the staff of the air desk at Aberdeen had even more options at their disposal.

During 1994 the Bölkow BO 105D operating from Inverness had increased its hours of cover from its initial eight hours a day, Monday to Friday, to ten hours a day, seven days a week. From April 1995 the Prestwick-based Bölkow BO 105D also increased its duty hours to this level.

Also operating the Bölkow BO 105 is Strathclyde Police. It is, only Scottish police force to operate an Air Support Unit, which was formed in November 1989. In the first five years of operation the Unit attended more than 14,000 incidents. A very small number of these were casevac (casualty evacuation) cases but the Unit's helicopter is equipped with a stretcher and fits happily into this emergency role when the need arises. Many of these have been life-threatening situations and indeed some of the injuries sustained by the patients ultimately resulted in their deaths following their arrival at hospital.

But Strathclyde Police have their success stories too. A climber injured after falling from the face of a Renfrewshire quarry, a two-week-old child who sustained injuries after a 70-foot fall in Dumbarton, and a paraglider pilot who was injured on 2,335-foot Tinto Hill in Lanarkshire are just some of the victims whose evacuations were successfully concluded.

The first flight of the Bölkow BO 105 took place in 1967 and it has continued to develop throughout the following quarter of a century. Now employed by ambulance services and police forces of many nations, it seems set to remain a familiar sight in its medevac and casevac role for many years yet to come.

In Scotland the patient has never been so well served. The remotest locations can be reached and casualty evacuations can be performed from the scenes of often diverse and horrific accidents. This has resulted in the transport of a greater number of patients by air and the saving of many more lives. It did not take long to prove that helicopter and fixed-wing aircraft could work in harmony, having their individual specialist attributes which could be put to the most appropriate use to fit the needs of a given situation. It is a formula that should endure into the next century.

The Second Column

The role of the Search and Rescue services

*T*HE DEPLOYMENT of helicopters for air ambulance flying is not a totally new idea in Scotland. The fixed-wing air ambulance service has for many years enjoyed the support of the Search and Rescue (SAR) services of the Royal Air Force, the Royal Navy, and more recently, of HM Coastguard, a role which is unlikely to diminish.

Indeed, as early as 1959, BEA was recording in its annual report that, 'An important development has been the linking of Service Helicopters with the air ambulance service. This has made it possible to extend this emergency medical service to islands without landing strips adequate for fixed-wing air ambulances.'

The RAF established its SAR operation in 1941. The need for such an organisation had been recognised because of the number of air crews having to ditch at sea during the early stages of the Second World War. During this period the luckier crews would launch a flotation dinghy from their disabled aircraft but they then had to await rescue by a vessel from a small and thinly-spread fleet of high speed launches. The resources available were totally inadequate as will be gleaned from the fact that between 10th and 30th July 1940 more than 200 aircrew were reported killed or missing, the majority of them over the sea.

The Directorate of Air/Sea Rescue Services took up its duties in February 1941. It was attached to Coastal Command and its duties did not only include co-ordination of searches; it also taught aircrews how to cope with a ditching at sea and how to survive until rescued, and it trained crews of rescue craft how to find ditched airmen and bring them home safely. The Directorate would use the Westland Lysander to locate aircrews in the water, drop a dinghy and ration pack, and mark their location with a smoke float. Supermarine Walrus amphibious aircraft then performed the actual rescue.

The first regular helicopter to be introduced by the SAR services was the Westland Dragonfly HR.3 which was based at RNAS Lossiemouth in 1952/53. On 2nd July 1956, one of these created a stir in Aberdeen when it made the first helicopter landing in the grounds of the Royal Infirmary. Its patient was a badly injured youth, 15-year-old Wilhelm Frederic Jansen, who had been plucked from the East German trawler *Gerhardt Zimmermann*, 90 miles out in the North Sea off Fraserburgh. The Dragonfly had lowered Surgeon-Lieutenant J Laine to the fishing vessel where he treated Jansen who was then hoisted up by the hovering helicopter in a wicker stretcher. Jansen's arm had been trapped in the trawler's winch and had to be amputated in Aberdeen Royal Infirmary that night but the rescue operation had saved his life. Because of the limitations in range and capacity of the Dragonfly, a second machine had accompanied it, with additional fuel, to Rosehearty. There the tanks of the first machine were replenished before it set out across the North Sea. And there was no room for Laine on the return journey. He eventually made it back to Aberdeen the following day aboard the *Gerhardt Zimmermann*.

This incident followed a major SAR operation on 3rd February of the same year when the Norwegian ship *Dovrefjell*, carrying 40 crew members, struck rocks in the Pentland Firth during a gale registering Force 9. Two Dragonflies from RNAS Lossiemouth and a Sycamore of 275 Squadron at RAF Leuchars performed the rescue. To achieve this they had to lift two men at a time and relay them to John O' Groats. The rescue lasted in excess of three hours. It was the first helicopter rescue at sea to be carried out on such a scale and it brought a stream of awards and citations to the airmen involved.

The RAF had chosen the Bristol Sycamore HR Mk.14 as its first SAR helicopter, but the arrival of the Sikorsky S-55 Whirlwind in 1955 was the signal of a massive step forward for the SAR services in their use of rotary aircraft and the increased versatility that helicopters put at their disposal. The Whirlwind was progressively developed, as the HAR.10 in the RAF and HAR.9 in the Royal Navy, continuing in use until 1981.

The capacity limitations of earlier helicopters was made quite explicit in a handbook issued to Highland General Practitioners who might have to call on the Services for air ambulance assistance. 'The chief differences, between the helicopters used by the Services, are of size. The Dragonfly, which is the smallest, is not big enough to take an adult stretcher patient enclosed; a stretcher protrudes from the sides, or in some cases may be completely outside the helicopter leaving the patient exposed. The Sycamore is larger and although an adult stretcher patient's legs would stick out beyond the fuselage, blister doors can be fitted so that the patient is completely enclosed, provided the canvas stretcher with detachable stretcher poles is used. The Whirlwind is, by helicopter standards, roomy and there is no difficulty in carrying two stretcher patients fully enclosed, and an attendant.'

The handbook, published in 1968, did offer some reassurance concerning patients exposed to the elements, advising that, on the Dragonfly, heating for the patient was provided by chemical hot water bottles while on the Sycamore an electric blanket was provided. The doctor was also expected to advise on a suitable landing site for the uplifting of his patient and was given instructions as to the area required and how it should be marked. 'It is helpful if the wind direction can be shown. This is best done by making smoke, well away from the touchdown point and not upwind of it, but a small fire or even a scarf held above the head will usually suffice.'

The doctor also had to ensure that spectators were kept clear and that the helicopter was approached with extreme caution. 'Special care must be taken when approaching a helicopter which has its engine running. The main danger is from the tail rotor which most people forget about and is difficult to see because of its high speed. The sweep of the main rotor also is low and could in certain circumstances easily hit a man's head. A blow from either would probably prove fatal and would ground the helicopter.'

Successor to the Whirlwind was the Westland Wessex HAR.2, still a familiar sight taking off with No. 22 Squadron at RAF Leuchars in the late 1980s. The Wessex excelled itself in rescues from mountains and cliff faces, a role which its successor, the Westland Sea King HAR.Mk.3, also performs with equal panache.

The scope of the RAF SAR service ranges far and wide and includes the scrambling of a Nimrod Mk.2P aircraft, from its base at RAF Kinloss, to the aid of vessels in distress. The Nimrod might remain airborne for seven hours, scanning the sea for wreckage or survivors and then co-ordinating rescue helicopters and sea vessels. In the aid of civilians, the SAR services of the RAF are particularly known for their helicopter operations in support of Mountain Rescue Teams. But their air ambulance involvement is by no means limited to this.

Flight Lieutenant Nick Stillwell operated from RAF Leuchars for two terms of duty, the first of these starting in 1980. 'In addition to mountain and sea rescue we would transfer patients between hospitals, assist at the scene of road accidents, and perform ambulance flights for the islands, particularly from locations some distance from an airfield and often at night or in bad weather. When the RAF SAR service was shared between Leuchars and Lossiemouth, we were performing between 150 and 200 civilian cases from each base annually.'

Dr Robert Martin had first hand experience of the Sea King in operation when an extremely ill diabetic patient had to taken from Oban to Edinburgh. 'At the time no aircraft of the Air Ambulance Service was available and the nearest aircraft was a Sea King which had just rescued a climber and taken him to Fort William for treatment. Flying this way was an experience as the pilot basically flew by roads and landmarks. At one point I was able to identify the summit of the Rest and be Thankful on the A82 which helped the pilot get his bearings. We flew into Edinburgh along the M8 motorway and then banked steeply above the capital which, with the door open, afforded quite a view. One of our oxygen cylinders slid towards the door only to be pulled up short as it was attached to the patient.'

The hazards that can be encountered by helicopter crews were illustrated to the full on 20th March 1989 when an RAF Sea King of 'D' Flight, under the command of John Prince, had to negotiate snow squalls to collect a meningitis patient from Broadford, Skye. The large helicopter had to make several field landings as heavy showers caused white-out conditions. The patient, Kirsteen Campbell, was eventually flown to Raigmore Hospital, Inverness, but she did not recover from the killer disease. The Sea King crew were quarantined for two days.

From Lossiemouth, 'D' Flight of the RAF's 202 Squadron operates two Sea King SAR helicopters in a role which it took over from British Airways Helicopters' Aberdeen-based Sikorsky S61N, and more recently from colleagues at RAF Leuchars and RAF Kinloss. In 1993 'D' Flight handled 214 civilian cases, culminating in December with its 3,000th mission since its Lossiemouth base was established 20 years earlier.

202 Squadron's aircraft are clearly identifiable because of their distinctive yellow livery. This provides an interesting litmus test of public perception. Civilian complaints about the noise generated by military aircraft are a fact of life but those registered against the SAR helicopters are proportionately lower than the average, indicating a greater level of public tolerance because of their life-saving activities. This has been proved on those occasions when a machine not carrying SAR colours has deputised for one of the regular machines. A sudden increase in noise complaints has immediately been recorded. A yellow Sea King apparently makes less noise than a blue Sea King.

Night Vision Goggles are a new aid at the disposal of each crew of 'D' Flight from 1994. These sophisticated pieces of apparatus, costing £15,000 per set, can rapidly increase the success of SAR missions in darkness because, by amplifying light 25,000 times, they can pick up the smallest glow in the dark from a small torch beam to the glow of a cigarette. One stranded climber in Glencoe called the rescue services on a mobile telephone who were then able to locate him quickly because of the backlighting on the phone.

Because of the popularity and the ruggedness of the terrain for which it is responsible, the Glencoe Mountain Rescue Team is one of Scotland's busiest. Cold statistics are often devoid of human drama but that is not the case when the Glencoe team's activities are reviewed. In 1993 the team attended 45 incidents which included 23 injured and 11 deaths. 3,684 man-hours were spent on the mountains responding to these call-outs and helicopters were used in 26 of these incidents.

Ronnie Rodger of the Glencoe Mountain Rescue Team is in no doubt about the value of the role played by the SAR services. 'Most of the people injured on the Glencoe mountains are flown to the Belford Hospital in Fort William by SAR helicopters. Seriously injured people are usually stabilised, then flown on to Raigmore Hospital in Inverness, or to one of the big city hospitals, such as the Southern General in Glasgow. I know that on many occasions these helicopters and their crews have saved lives.'

The RAF maintains Mountain Rescue Teams of its own at Kinloss and Leuchars. Each team has four or five full-time leaders but the remainder of the 35 men, who make up each team, are volunteers. In addition to helping in the search for missing or injured climbers, the teams have assisted in the hunt for missing children and have been at the scene of major disasters such as that caused by the crash of a Pan Am Boeing 747 at Lockerbie on the night of 20th December 1988.

RAF Boulmer in Northumberland is the headquarters of 202 Squadron. Its close proximity to the Scottish border means that SAR missions to the Southern Uplands are frequently operated from that station.

At Prestwick the Royal Navy's 819 Squadron at *HMS Gannet* operates the Sea King HAS.6, replacing earlier versions from 1989. The station occupies Greensite which, in 1952, was created to the north of the airport as a United States Air Force Search & Rescue base. The USAF moved on in 1966 and, following major reconstruction, the site became *HMS Gannet* in 1971. 819 Squadron arrived in October of the same year.

Lt Angus Paterson recalls a couple of early offshore rescues. 'The Sea King's superior endurance and improved transit speeds, when compared to those of its predecessor, made it an ideal long range Search and Rescue asset. An incident worthy of note was the rescue of a Russian fisherman from the trawler *Taras Shevenko* off Rockall on 24 June 1974, at the height of the Cold War. This proved to be quite a feat considering the distances involved (700 nautical miles round trip) and the logistics of long range SAR which were still in their infancy. The Sea King had established itself as an invaluable vehicle and continued to be tasked in the role. The salvage capability of the aircraft was put to the test on 2nd August 1974 when 819 Squadron was tasked to lift a stricken hovercraft that had run aground on Ardmore Point following an engine failure.'

819's Sea Kings were tested to their limits on 2nd November 1982 when two machines were called to the assistance of the fishing boat *Poseidon*, in a raging storm, north of the Isle of Skye. Other fishing boats standing by watched *Poseidon*'s situation deteriorate as it foundered on the rocks of Fladda Chuain and its crew took to the water. Flying blind into rain and seaspray, the helicopters were guided by flares from the other vessels to a point where the fishermen could be winched up, and snatched from certain death. The operation lasted seven hours.

On 11th January 1986, the Squadron's Sea King was refuelling at Benbecula having been out earlier to a vessel in distress, when the Rescue Co-ordination Centre at Pitreavie received a call to uplift the victim of a road accident on the Isle of Mull. The Sea King lifted off at 9.00pm, flying into winds gusting at 70 knots, to land in a field at Glenforsa, illuminated by the headlights of a police vehicle. The woman casualty's leg had been severed, necessitating urgent departure to Glasgow Airport and the Southern General Hospital where emergency surgery enabled the leg to be restored to its proper place.

A medevac operation occurred in January 1987 in an uncharacteristically urban environment when 11-year-old Claire Moncur, with suspected meningitis, had to be uplifted from Avonhead, two miles north of Caldercruix in Lanarkshire, and flown to hospital in Glasgow. Heavy snowfalls, with drifts 6 feet in height, had prevented a doctor from reaching the girl's home for several days. In desperation, the girl's mother had contacted the police who, in a combined effort with prison officers and inmates from nearby Longriggend Remand Centre, saw the creation of an impromptu landing area for the Sea King near the family's cottage.

Captain Don Henry was in command of the Sea King and he experienced worsening conditions as he flew inland from Prestwick. 'Visibility was bad and we had to fly low and follow the roads until we saw the officers waving at us. Landing was also difficult because the snow made it hard to judge the slope of the ground.' Don flew Claire, accompanied by her father, to Glasgow's Southern General, only to find high winds making a landing in a confined space extremely dangerous. The only option was to continue on to Glasgow Airport where a road ambulance would take over. Road conditions west of Glasgow were less extreme than those left behind in Lanarkshire but it took the ambulance three times as long as normal to make the journey from the airport to the city. Claire later made a full recovery.

819 Squadron's primary function is an anti-submarine role but, since 1975, it has had a SAR helicopter on permanent 90-minute standby by night or 45 minutes by day. In 1989 these times were reduced to 45 and 15 minutes, respectively. Between 1975 and 1981 the squadron attended more than 300 incidents but by 1993 the Squadron was responding to 230 call-outs in that single year. Of these, 99 were medevac cases, compared with 47 in 1992, reflecting the increased demand experienced from Kintyre and the Hebrides during the initial period when Scottish Air Ambulance duties were transferred from fixed-wing aircraft to Bölkow BO 105 helicopters operating restricted hours.

819 Naval Air Squadron has approximately 100 engineers maintaining its fleet of Sea Kings and it can call on men and women, who serve as medical attendants at the station's Sick Bay, to join a SAR crew within a matter of minutes. Unlike its RAF counterpart at Lossiemouth, this Squadron does not have aircraft dedicated to the SAR role. New Zealander Neill Stephenson is one of the pilots on regular SAR standby duty, 'We can normally carry two stretchers with additional seating for a couple of relatives or a doctor if we feel it necessary to have one in attendance. Space in the rear of the aircraft also accommodates two medical attendants who can administer first aid and operate the winch, and the radar operator whose array of sophisticated equipment is installed for the primary duties of the Squadron, anti-submarine defence. While SAR is a secondary activity for the Squadron, this role provides valuable training, often involving flying over difficult terrain in adverse conditions, while simultaneously providing a life-saving service.'

By far the most traumatic year for the Squadron was 1988, when it provided several crews to assist in the North Sea following the Piper Alpha oil platform explosion on 6th July, resulting in more than 160 fatalities. On 20th December of the same year 819 Squadron helicopters were quickly at Lockerbie along with those of their RAF colleagues, following the mid-air explosion of the Pan American Boeing 747 which resulted in 270 deaths.

The normal area covered by Prestwick-based 819 Squadron for Search and Rescue missions has its aircraft heading seaward to the west up to a range of 200 miles or landward as far north as Fort William.

The Rescue Co-ordination Centre at Pitreavie Castle, Dunfermline, co-ordinates SAR operations in Scotland. The SAR services of the RAF and of the Royal Navy were originally established to provide a rescue service for the crews of the Services' own aircraft. Yet such rescues now account for less than 5 percent of the hundreds of people who are assisted annually. The Search and Rescue roles of the RAF and Royal Navy are of paramount importance in Scotland. The islands, the mountains, the isolation all militate against rapid surface transport.

It is HM Coastguard which provides SAR cover from bases in the islands with units located at Sumburgh and Stornoway. The Stornoway Coastguard SAR helicopter. operated by Bristow Aviation's Sikorsky S61N G-BIMU *Loch Fyne*, began operations on 12th May 1987. In December 1985 six crewmen from the fishing vessel *Bon Ami* died when the boat ran aground on the north-west coast. This incident highlighted a need for SAR services to be available for a quick response in this area and the establishing of the Coastguard's SAR station at Stornoway stemmed directly from the assessments which followed. When its large Sikorsky S61N flew Norman Finlayson (who had fallen from a ladder at his home in Ness on the Isle of Lewis) from Stornoway to Glasgow's Southern General Hospital in August 1991, it marked the unit's 500th mission.

At Sumburgh the HM Coastguard contract is operated by Bristow's Sikorsky S61N G-BDOC *Tolquhoun*, a 24-hour dedicated SAR service that spawned from a service begun on 1st November 1971 with BEA Helicopters operating a S61N on behalf of the Coastguard at Aberdeen. After some years the contract transferred from Aberdeen to Sumburgh, by which time BEA Helicopters had been renamed British Airways Helicopters. In 1983 the contract passed to Bristow Helicopters.

Bristow's Shetland SAR crew have been called upon to assist at several major maritime incidents involving large numbers of casualties. 'Oscar Charlie' flew for nearly 26 hours, with four crew changes, during the Piper Alpha disaster. And on 9th November 1993, in relays, she lifted a total of 56 crewmen from the Latvian fish factory ship *Lunoholds* when it was blown on to the rocks below the cliffs of the Isle of Bressay. During this rescue Winchman Friedie Manson had to cope with rigging and infrastructure on the vessel while it was being regularly engulfed by massive waves.

Unlike its cousin, the Sea King, the Sikorsky S61N is extremely spacious with a large 'work area' where casualties can be winched aboard and then attended by the medical staff. It can comfortably carry three stretchers, incubators, and other medical equipment. An ample seating area in the rear of the aircraft can accommodate relatives and medical staff. With these seats removed, stretcher space can be provided for as many as ten patients.

The aircraft carries distinctive colours, but fishing vessels in difficulty have been known to give its arrival a mixed response. This is because their crews can see the large lettering 'HM Coastguard' on the side before they notice the small 'Search and Rescue' titles under the nose and, if of a nervous disposition, they sometimes presume that the helicopter is descending to monitor their fishing activities rather than to aid an ill or injured crew member.

A staff of 21 operates the Bristow contract for HM Coastguard at Stornoway, including three engineers to maintain the helicopter. A crew consisting of two pilots, a winchman, and a winch operator, is constantly standing by in the crew room at Stornoway Airport. A piece of broken rotor from a helicopter, which in 1988 ditched in the sea, decorates the duty room wall as a reminder of the constant hazards being faced. The two crewmen at the winch are trained in first aid but when this large expensive machine is employed in medevac cases it is usually because they are extremely serious and an appropriately experienced nurse, doctor, or specialist will accompany the patient. A list of medical personnel on Lewis is maintained so that the appropriate staff can be called out at short notice.

A doctor requiring a medical evacuation initially makes contact with the Scottish Ambulance Service in Aberdeen where the centre will call HM Coastguard in Stornoway if it considers that it will be most suitably equipped to carry the case. HM Coastguard, from its nerve centre at Battery Point overlooking Stornoway Harbour, will then instruct the Bristow crew to respond to the call.

Nearly a quarter of the Coastguard flights are for medevacs and most of these are for transfers between hospitals, from the Outer Hebrides to the mainland or from Daliburgh Hospital on South Uist to Stornoway. For what the crews nickname 'Pregevacs', a midwife or Consultant Obstetrician will often accompany the patient or there will be a Consultant Paediatrician to assist with incubator cases. Midwives are regularly brought to Stornoway Airport for familiarisation with the Sikorsky S61N.

Captain Roger Asbey has been at Stornoway since 1987. Concentrating on the front end, he usually sees medical cases only as 'a bundle of blankets with a head sticking out'. But he has become extremely familiar with the western seaboard of Scotland and points out that his territory, which runs from Oban to Cape Wrath, 'would cross the Atlantic if it were laid out in a straight line'.

Simon Riley of Stornoway Coastguard explains the delicate balancing act required when tasking the Sikorsky S61N. 'The helicopter's primary function is assisting with maritime incidents. We therefore have to be extremely careful when responding to medevac requests. These are often because of poor weather conditions. Therefore we get a bit nervous when asked to send the helicopter "out of area" to points such as Glasgow. Even Inverness can be a problem because, if the weather is bad, the pilot might be unable to cross the mountains and have to follow the Sutherland coast. If the weather at Inverness is likely to present problems, it has not been unknown for a helicopter to have to refuel in *Aberdeen* while flying the long way round from Stornoway to Inverness (Stornoway-Cape Wrath-Caithness-Aberdeen fuel stop-Inverness). It would obviously be very embarrassing if we were unable to use our own helicopter to answer a maritime emergency because it was two hours away transferring a patient to a Glasgow hospital. But we enjoy good teamwork and with co-operation all round we have a system which works well.'

The maritime area covered by the helicopter takes it over the Atlantic to Rockall, that barren pinpoint of isolated rock in the west, and to the Faroe Islands well to the north. Simon Riley explains, 'G-BIMU is fitted with long-range fuel tanks but Rockall takes us to the limit. The Nimrod long range reconnaissance aircraft of RAF Lossiemouth plays an invaluable role in these extremities as we rely on them to pinpoint a vessel in distress so that we can fly directly to the scene, allow ten minutes to winch up sea crew in distress, and head straight back for landfall, usually Benbecula.'

Maritime rescues and assistance are defined as including islands and lighthouses which do not have ship landing facilities. While most lighthouses are now unmanned, they are visited by maintenance engineers who, by the nature of their work, are exposed to some risk in isolated situations.

The Coastguard helicopter carries infra-red detection equipment, permitting it to operate at night and in poor visibility. One rescue using this equipment saved two people from certain death. The couple had taken a walk along the base of cliffs near Applecross in Wester Ross only to be caught by the tide on a cliff ledge as they emerged from a cave. Cold and wet, they were trapped on the face of the cliff with darkness falling. As the night wore on, a search was mounted for the walkers in vain and the Stornoway helicopter was called to assist.

Winchman Terry Freeman recalls what happened next. 'It was nearly 3.00am and the outside temperature was zero. There was a high wind and a big swell. I switched on the FLIR (Forward Looking Infra-Red) and, during our first run along the cliff, I noticed two bright dots on the screen. There were other sources of heat in view — sheep on the hilltop — but they were moving about. I marked the spot and the pilot turned out to sea to make

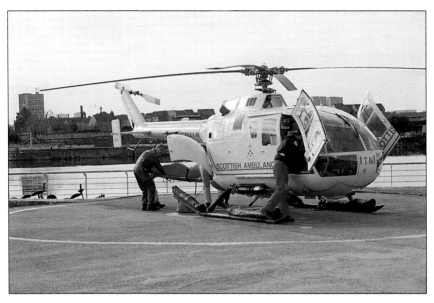

Prestwick-based Bölkow BO 105D at the Glasgow city helipad in 1993.
(Photo by Stuart G Sim)

Bond Helicopters' air ambulance base at Inverness Airport.
(Photo by the author)

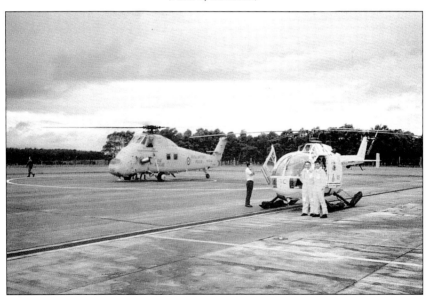

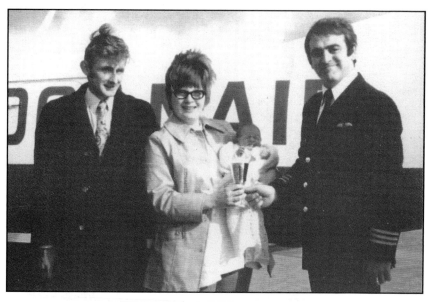

Charles and Freida Devin accept an inscribed goblet
from Captain Jamie Bayley at Kirkwall Airport on 8th August 1973
to mark the birth of Katy, Loganair's first inflight baby.
(Photo courtesy of Loganair)

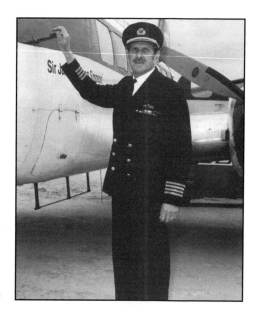

Captain Eric Starling,
BEA Flight Manager 1947-1968,
and Air Ambulance Captain 1968-1971.
(Photo courtesy of Tony Naylor)

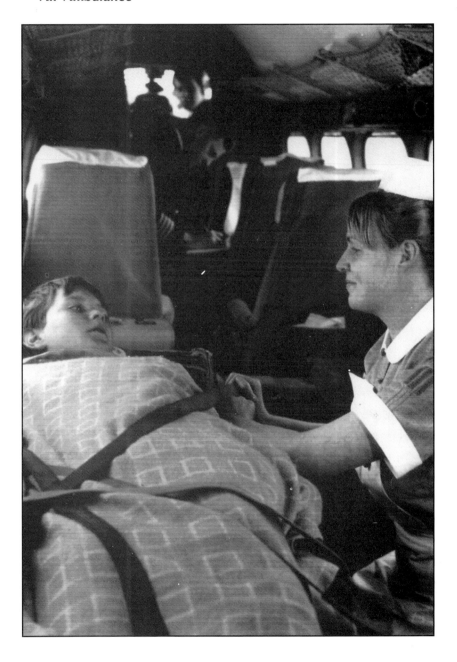

Words of comfort to a young patient on the Heron.
(Photo BEA, courtesy of Captain Ian Montgomery)

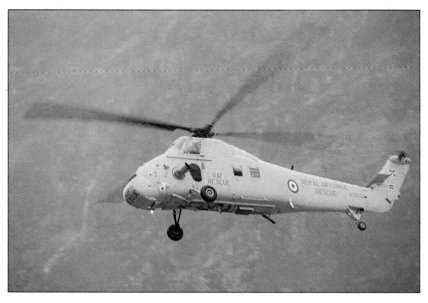

Westland Wessex of the RAF SAR in Glencoe in 1987.
(Photo by the author)

RAF Westland Sea King in Glencoe, also in 1987.
(Photo by the author)

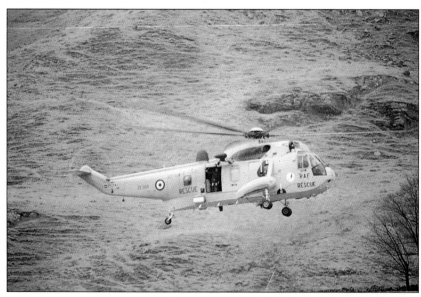

a fresh approach. The couple must have thought we were leaving them but they showed up so well on the screen, we couldn't have missed them.' The walkers were winched to safety after spending ten hours on the cliff face.

On 2nd April 1989 the Stornoway Coastguard helicopter was flying over Loch Erisort on the Isle of Lewis when the passenger manifest increased by one. Catherine Macleod of Locheport was being flown from her North Uist home to Stornoway to give birth. But baby Kirsty saw an opportunity for her name to appear in the record books and as she was not about to pass it up she arrived mid-flight.

For Winchman Tab Hunter, this was his introduction to Stornoway Coastguard SAR flying, and what a first flight. 'I assured the midwife that everything would be fine as we were only ten minutes' flying time from Stornoway. But she was in no doubt that the baby was not going to hold on for another ten minutes.'

The helicopter crew presented Kirsty with a silver christening cup engraved with a map showing the location of her birth, and a framed photograph of the helicopter in which the event took place. Her mother was showered with flowers while her father, art teacher Donald Macleod, must have found the gift of a bottle of malt whisky very acceptable. His painting of G-BIMU in flight, now hanging in the Bristow duty room at Stornoway Airport, is testament to Donald Macleod's return gesture.

Coastguard helicopter crews are regularly hailed for their bravery although to them it is all part of the job. One of many examples cited for a Commendation for Meritorious Service by the Chief Coastguard reads, 'On 27th November 1991, for the successful evacuation of the crew of the fishing vessel *Baruth* 20 miles west of the Isle of Scarp, NW Scotland. When the *Baruth* reported that she was taking water during appalling weather conditions, HM Coastguard SAR helicopter under the command of Captain Roger Asbey was scrambled to evacuate the crew. In severe gale Force 9 winds and with the vessel rolling heavily in a 20 ft swell, the crew of the helicopter displayed outstanding skill and airmanship of a high order in ensuring the safe evacuation of the fishing vessel's crew of 6. During the rescue, the helicopter winchman, Tab Hunter, was struck by the rolling vessel and severely bruised in the ribs, yet continued with the mission despite his injury.'

The Doctors Macleod
Lochmaddy
by
Dr John A J Macleod

'Clach air an charn.'

'A stone on their cairn.'

To the memory of my parents
Dr Alex J Macleod and Dr Julia P Macleod

*D*R ALEX J MACLEOD OBE FRCGP (1894-1979), ably assisted by his wife Dr Julia P Macleod MB ChB (1901-1992), was the Medical Practitioner for the islands of North Uist and Berneray from 1932 to 1974. In 1973 he was joined by his son Dr John A J Macleod DL FRCGP who has continued in the Practice and maintained the family interest in the air ambulance service. Dr Alex J Macleod was the first doctor to use an aircraft to move a patient in the Outer Hebrides (22 May 1933) and for the rest of his working and retired life fought for the continued improvement of the service.

First Outer Hebrides Flight

During May 1933, my father, Dr A J Macleod, was returning from a (rare at that time) post-graduate medical course at Cambridge. While passing through Glasgow he went to the Western Infirmary to visit one of his patients, the Rev Malcolm Gillies of Clachan Church, North Uist. He found that the man was so ill that the hospital staff felt that he would not survive a homeward journey by train and boat and so they were preparing to continue his terminal care in Glasgow.

Rev Gillies was weak but was able to speak and he was desperate to return home to die in his own manse, among his own parishioners and with his wife caring for him. My father had seen the press accounts of the evacuation from Islay of John McDermid on 14th May 1933 so he set about trying to find an aircraft and a sponsor to bring the Rev Gillies home. Agreement was reached for the use of a de Havilland DH84 Dragon, which was one of two that had newly arrived at Renfrew Airport for Midland & Scottish Air Ferries, and the *Daily Record* paid for the trip. Captain Jimmy Orrell was the pilot and the flight was reported in the *Daily Record* and other newspapers next day.

Father had clear knowledge of the tides and was able to give a suitable time for landing on the firm sand about 700 yards from the manse. He sent various telegrams to North Uist warning people to be ready with horse and cart for the final stage of the trip. Rev Gillies survived until September 1933 and was so pleased that he was able to spend his last months at home. It all went successfully and this was the first time that an aircraft had been used for the transport of a patient in the Outer Hebrides. It also established, for the future service, that bringing home an invalid *from* hospital was as much a part of the service as taking an ill person to hospital.

The flight is now being commemorated by North Uist Community Council which is erecting a plaque by the main road (A865) close to the landing site. The place where the aircraft landed is tidal and it lies to the west of Clachan Church and to the south of the Mermaid Fish Shop. This first Outer Hebridean ambulance flight also marked the start of a long and close relationship between the Macleod family and the pilots and nurses of the Air Ambulance Service.

The Early Years

The early landings on North Uist were made on various stretches of tidal beach. Once the formal grass strip was opened at Sollas in 1936, most flights operated from there, although, as late as 1959, before the North Ford causeway had been completed, there was an evacuation from the beach at Grimsay.

The use of aircraft brought a new dimension into the management of sick people in isolated island communities; and having been the first doctor to use an aircraft in the Outer Hebrides, my father continued to push for developments in and improvements to the service. By his regular contact with the pilots he was continually aware of advances in aviation and from the mid-sixties until his death in 1979, he constantly tried to have the service upgraded by having a helicopter stationed in the islands. He saw the difficulties that the RAF helicopters of the time had in crossing the high ground from the east to the west of the Highlands and he would have been delighted to know that a Coastguard helicopter is now stationed at Stornoway. It has a major role in the moving of ambulance cases, particularly on occasions when a fixed-wing aircraft cannot fly or if the patient is in a difficult place for removal.

In the early years, arranging a flight was very difficult as there were no telephones on North Uist and contact with the mainland had to be by telegram. Particularly during the 1939-45 period there were restrictions on that limited service and so special 'Priority' telegraph request forms were issued to island doctors. In 1943 they had to send these to 'Gunn, Health, Edinburgh'.

A senior civil servant in the Department of Health then arranged the flight through the Air Ministry. There were also great difficulties with communications within the island as, once he had seen the patient, my father would have to drive back to the surgery to send the message and then wait for the reply.

When I was aged about nine I caused a bit of chaos in that I messed up one of these telegraphic requests for an aircraft. I had walked the mile home from school for lunch and, as I would be passing the Post Office on my return to school, I was given one of these special Priority Telegram forms to hand in. It seems that I lost it and either forgot about it or, more likely, was too afraid to say anything about it because after some hours another telegram was sent. A few days later the original was found in a roadside ditch!

In 1943 the film *Highland Doctor* was made by the Ministry of Information in order to portray the work of the Highlands and Islands medical scheme. The film was shown throughout the UK to illustrate the benefits of an existing form of State Health Scheme and show that the proposed National Health Service would be good for everyone. The section on the Air Ambulance was based on my father and his work. Actors were used to portray a specialist coming by the thrice-weekly steamer, meeting the local doctor, driving to see the patient and then deciding that the patient should be flown to hospital by air ambulance. The Rapide arrived and, for the sake of the film, landed on the sand, even though the formal grass strip at Sollas was only a mile away. Father was not in the film but was on hand over the two days of filming to advise the producer, actors and the film crew.

The benefits of the air ambulance service to the isolated doctor and his patients were of course immense. The man whose stomach ulcer burst while he was sowing seed on the offshore island of Baleshare was lifted from the adjacent sandy beach by David Barclay on 30th June 1937. Many years later, on the island of Vallay off the north shore of North Uist, a man had a leg badly smashed when he fell under his horse and cart and he was also lifted from the sandy beach.

Although most pregnant women had their babies on the island, some had to be flown out with the development of complications in early labour. In one such incident the baby was born in the aircraft and although there was an existing statute for babies being born at sea in that they were registered at the first UK port reached, no such statute then existed for babies born in the air. The pilot had to estimate his position at the time of birth and so there was an occasion when a North Uist father had to spend six days travelling by steamer and train to register the new arrival with the Registrar of Births in Lochgilphead which had been the nearest Registry Office to the location of birth.

It also became possible for a medical specialist to fly in and either manage the expectant mother at home or load her on to the waiting aircraft. The late Sir Hector Maclennan (Obstetrician, Glasgow) once hurriedly left his hospital clinic and arrived in his city suit and shiny black shoes to advise on a lady who had developed a dangerous complication of her pregnancy. He assessed her as being fit to travel and, as her husband was keen to go with her, he stayed behind on the island.

It was a nasty day but he insisted in joining the local men who were holding down the wings of the Rapide during take-off from a nearby beach. His suit and shoes were ruined and his black Homburg hat went bouncing away through the salty water. It was later recovered a mile away and found its way back to Glasgow even though it was no longer fit for wearing in the city. Sir Hector's son, Robert Maclennan MP, was later to be a great help to my father when he was pushing for helicopters.

Although ambulance flights were initially used for fairly dramatic situations, their use was gradually extended to include those patients, going for elective operations, who would have had difficulty either travelling by ferry and train or by the scheduled aircraft. Sometimes two or three patients in this category would be gathered together and a flight arranged for later in the week.

The number of mothers going to mainland hospitals for the delivery of their babies increased and, as there was an IATA rule prohibiting the carriage of a pregnant passenger by scheduled flight after the 36th week of confinement, the air ambulance was used to carry them. At the time when this rule was being rigorously enforced, BEA was running the scheduled flights from Benbecula and had the contract for the air ambulance. I have seen the Heron land at Benbecula to pick up a woman, who was fit but in her 37th week of pregnancy, and park alongside the BEA Viscount operating the scheduled service. Later the rule was amended for scheduled flights operating internal UK routes and now pregnant mothers can fly up to the end of the 38th week which is far more sensible.

The Monach Isles

The Monach Isles are a group of low sandy islands about seven miles west of North Uist and there was a tall lighthouse on Shillay which had a tidal link with Ceann Iar.

The majority of the families who had lived on the Monachs had left in 1935 but some remained until 1942. Some of the others returned at intervals to deal with the sheep and cattle that were still kept there or for lobster fishing. During 1939 one of the lighthouse keepers on Shillay had his daughter staying with him on holiday. She became unwell with abdominal pain which was later found to be caused by appendicitis. A call was made via the lighthouse radio and it was picked up by the radio station at Sollas (North Uist) airport which at that time was the centre of Hebridean flying and the base for the schedule aircraft. The pilot was the New Zealander John Hankins, who lived at that time on North Uist in order to operate the air service.

Hank had previously made a trial landing on the Monachs so, instead of my father going out by the boat as would be usual, Hank volunteered to take him out and also to take the patient off if required. It was a westerly breeze and this was different from the time of his previous landing. He was just able to land. My father saw the patient at the lighthouse cottage and she was brought over to Ceann Iar by boat.

The added weight of the patient and her father now created a new problem as take-off with the wind from the west did not seem possible. Luckily there were several men there that day so they got busy filling in hollows and levelling ground opposite one of the natural features of any sand dunes, the 'blow hole'. This is a gap where the wind has caused a break in the bank above the shore.

One side of the blow hole was dug away to make it wider and then the aircraft was pushed into position down wind of the blow hole and down a slight slope. With a very short run over rough ground, Hank took off uphill through the gap and used the uplift of the wind coming through the blow hole to become airborne. This was a technique similar to that which, in modern times, is used on aircraft carriers for jet fighters to take off from a short deck. Hank landed at Sollas to top up with fuel and drop off my father, then continued to Glasgow where the patient had a successful operation.

The Committee Road

An aircraft approaching North Uist from the south in misty conditions could use the navigational aids at Benbecula Airport to reach that far but the pilot had to fly visually after that. By flying low and heading north from Benbecula the pilot could follow the coast of North Uist but then the mist would be a wall over the small hills in the middle of the island.

He then had to pick up the west end of a small twisty road that ran in a valley across North Uist and this took him out at Sollas, just near the landing strip. This was the 'Committee Road' and it was a welcome navigational aid in misty weather. It is so called because it was built at a time of famine by the Committee for the Relief of the Destitute and Poor.

Once the civilian airfield at Sollas closed, the Committee Road became even more important as an aid. When BEA introduced the Pionair (a converted Dakota) for the service flight to Benbecula, scheduled flights by the Rapide to Sollas ended. The grass strip at Sollas remained usable for a few years but then it was returned to active crofting use and was ploughed. The beach was then used until the North Ford Causeway opened in 1960 but only upon one or two occasions after that.

During the time after the Sollas base had closed, but while the strip was still usable, no fuel was available. So if the aircraft had brought a patient back from hospital and was taking another one out, the pilot had to fly to Benbecula to refuel and then return for the outward bound patient. I remember once taking that short trip with David Barclay. It was a southerly breeze so instead of using the landing strip for take-off, he ran up a small knoll on the north of the strip, turned and, with only a short run, was into the air. While passing over the Committee Road he had me lean over his shoulder and take the controls . . . a great thrill for a small boy.

When David Barclay retired on 30th April 1965, many presentations were made to him and his wife Nina from within BEA and from many grateful passengers and patients throughout the islands. On 29th April he made an air ambulance flight from Shetland to Aberdeen and then on 30th April his final trip was with the Heron for the scheduled run to Tiree and Barra. His younger daughter, Patricia, was a BEA stewardess based in Jersey and the company arranged for her to come north and fly with him on his last trip. At Tiree and Barra well-wishers were there to welcome him, bearing many and varied gifts for the veteran flyer of the Western Isles.

On 7th December 1965, my father organised a special presentation ceremony and cèilidh in North Uist. Money had been gathered by the District Council and the people of North Uist and Berneray had given generously. David and Nina Barclay were escorted on the trip by Captain Eric Starling and, to his surprise, there were also gifts for him and his wife Eleanor who had been unable to travel to the island. When they flew back to Glasgow they took with them a leg of prime North Uist heather-fed lamb which was for Captain Donald Hoare who had helped to arrange the trip and had also been responsible for ensuring that Captain Starling came along.

Low Flying

Early flying tended to be at low level and for some areas the pilot would use a road map or an Ordnance Survey map rather than an 'Air Map'. Those pilots got to know the shape of the Scottish coastline and of the individual islands so well that a brief gap in cloud or fog was enough for them to identify or locate an accurate position. With the introduction of more sophisticated navigational aids the planes flew higher and this started to create problems for some patients.

Patients with heart or lung failure or with certain bowel problems became quite unwell during the flights and giving oxygen to them by mask did not help a lot. This was because of the drop in atmospheric pressure at altitude, gas in the bowel expanding, and so pressure was put on other organs. In the case of a stomach ulcer that had been bleeding, this expansion could cause the clot to be stretched; bleeding would start again and the nurse would have to work hard to keep the patient alive.

In 1965 Captain Pat Eadie came to Glasgow to join the Heron team. At home, in New Zealand, he had done a lot of low flying and one of the special jobs that he had undertaken involved flying low to photograph construction schemes in isolated places. Serial photographs gave the company engineers a new way of assessing progress on their distant sites.

Following a couple of instances where patients' conditions had become worse at normal flying levels, Pat Eadie decided to work out low level routes to Glasgow from each island. He had several discussions with the now retired David Barclay and borrowed some of his old maps. The low level route from the Uists involved going round Mull instead of over it, crossing Kintyre by following the Crinan Canal and then staying near sea level down Loch Fyne and up the estuary of the River Clyde. When he was flying the scheduled routes to Barra or Islay he would practise on these routes. Passengers loved this but he was continually taken to task by Air Traffic Control as they could not track him at such low altitudes.

Carpetted

In 1949 the emerging National Health Service was feeling its way and the islands were being administered from Inverness. Doctors in official positions there took exception to a doctor in the islands using an aircraft for anything other than what they considered to be a dire emergency. Instead of arranging to meet him to discuss what were really confidential patient details, they launched an attack on Father's work via a routine Health Committee meeting at Inverness.

The press loved this and initially produced some juicy headlines, unfavourable to my father. But once the correspondents had been out to the islands to find out more details, they became very supportive and it ended with the press chiding the Inverness bosses for not having themselves gone out to learn at first hand some data on the fine work that was being done on North Uist and how much patients were benefitting. This episode served to confirm that it was the doctor on the spot who should decide when and for what kind of patient an aircraft was to be used, rather than have his or her fate dictated by a committee or its representative in an office on the other side of Scotland.

In the mid-fifties there was another attack on Father from officialdom in Inverness. This time it was the all-powerful Medical Officer of Health (MOH) who took exception to Uist patients being taken to Glasgow hospitals when he felt they should have been taken to Raigmore Hospital at Inverness.

Again the first word of this onslaught was via the press and again it became supportive when they received Father's terse explanatory response to their reporters. They were informed that (1) the aircraft and crew were based at Glasgow and should be back there as soon as possible; (2) in bad weather, flights between Uist and Glasgow were far easier than between Uist and Inverness, where the Highland mountains caused problems; (3) Uist people had relatives and friends in Glasgow but rarely in Inverness; and (4) the referring doctor was the one to decide what form of further care was necessary.

This confrontation confirmed that the island doctor could choose the hospital into which his patient would be admitted and this principle was not challenged again for more than thirty years until the management of the service was handed over to the Scottish Ambulance Service in 1993 and it initially tried to suggest that their duty officer would be the best person to decide to which hospital a patient should be delivered.

The Macleod Basket

Pilots' hours were not so rigorously adhered to in the early years, so quite often a pilot returning to Glasgow from a scheduled flight would find that he had to turn round rapidly. There would only be time for a quick weather briefing before he was gathering up the flight kit and a waiting nurse and heading back out to the islands. There would be no time in these circumstances for the pilot and his radio operator to have the meal that they might have been expecting.

From this arose the famous Macleod Basket, a welcome container which was packed tight with coffee, tea and sandwiches and taken to the landing site. The air-crew and nurse would sit in the car on the edge of the beach or grass strip and eat up the food of the day. Mutton sandwiches were very popular with the crews but this created a problem on Fridays as one of the Radio Officers, Hugh McGinlay, a Roman Catholic, did not eat meat on Fridays. An attempt was always made to find out if he would be on the flight and an alternative type of sandwich would be ready.

Even after the opening of the causeway to Benbecula in 1960, resulting in flights landing there rather than on North Uist, the Basket tradition continued but with the sandwiches being eaten in the comfort of the small terminal building. The tradition has now lapsed with the increase in the use of the service and the requirement that the aircraft turn around as fast as possible to return to base. The flight crews are on rota and do not suffer the same hunger pangs as in the past.

The Basket still exists and in 1993, when Captain Bill Innes was researching his programme about the early years of flying for Gaelic Television, many of the pilots to whom he spoke commented on it. He came to Lochmaddy in 1994 to take photographs of the famous Basket and reminded us of the many times when he was flying in the Heron fleet that he had welcomed the coffee and sandwiches from it.

The Crash

In the early hours of Saturday 28th September 1957, the only crash to result in fatalities occurred. Captain Paddy Calderwood had taken off in a Heron from Renfrew in bad weather to collect a seriously ill lady from the island of Islay. The weather turned out to be even worse there and, in turning to land, a wing tip hit the ground. Captain Calderwood, Radio

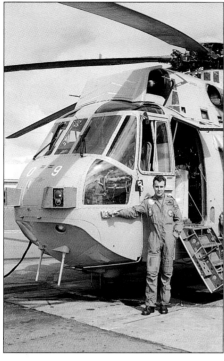

New Zealander Neill Stephenson is one of 819 Squadron's Sea King pilots at Prestwick.
(Photo by the author)

Sea King of the Royal Navy's 819 Squadron at Prestwick, 1994.
(Photo by the author)

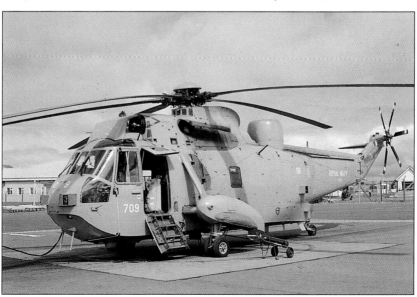

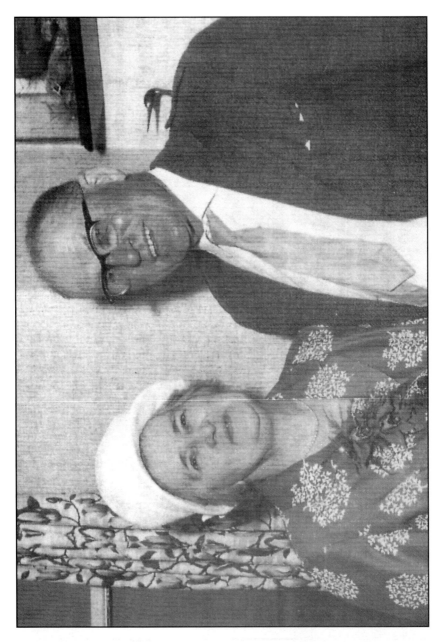

Dr Julia P Macleod and Dr Alex J Macleod of Lochmaddy, April 1965.
(Photo courtesy of Dr John A J Macleod)

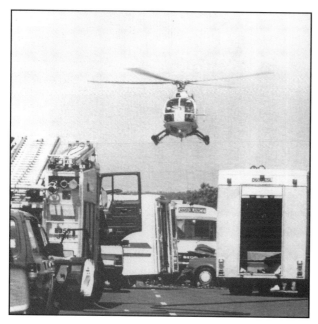

The First Air helicopter experiment is put to the test during a 1988 road accident.
(Photo courtesy of Scottish Ambulance Service)

(Below) Paramedics Robert Devine and Gerry Kelly attend a patient on a mountainside while Captain Phil Green phones ahead with an update on the progress of the evacuation.
(Photo courtesy of Scottish Ambulance Service)

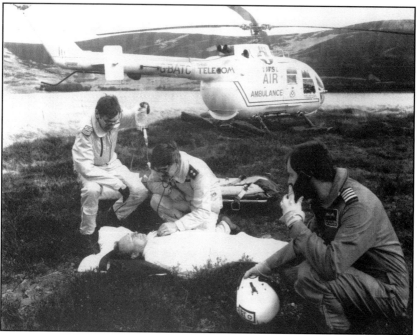

The spacious interior of the HM
Coastguard SAR Sikorsky S61N.
(Photo by the author)

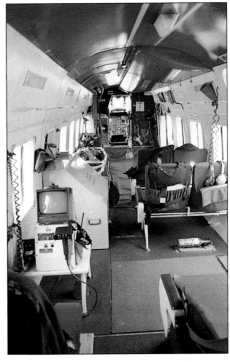

Bristow Sikorsky S61N G-BIMU on
standby for HM Coastguard at
Stornoway, 1994.
(Photo by the author)

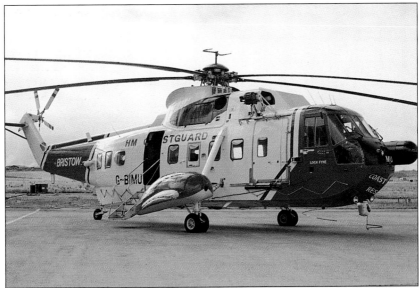

Officer Hugh McGinlay and Nursing Sister Jean Kennedy were all killed. The Civil Aviation Investigator, Mr W H Tench stated, 'It is obvious that the pilot was determined to do everything possible to save a desperately ill woman. He went to the uttermost limits to bring the plane in.'

Captain Eric Starling, as Flight Manager, then flew from Renfrew in a second Heron to collect the patient. Unfortunately she died in the plane on the way back to Renfrew.

I find it truly amazing that there had been no previous accidents. The earlier aircraft were simple and navigational aids were basic. The fact that there had not been an accident until that time — 24 years of year-round flying in sometimes appalling conditions — is a tribute to the skills of the pilots and to their knowledge of the west of Scotland and the islands.

Up to this point, in times of bad weather, the duty manager would explain to the pilot that the conditions were beyond company limits and the pilot then would decide whether or not he would fly. Tighter flight rules were then drawn up, and in the seventies, on ringing for an aeroplane, the duty officer would sometimes say that a flight was not going to be possible for some hours. Also in the 'sixties and 'seventies there were occasions when a fixed-wing aircraft could not fly and even the RAF helicopter could not fly over the Highland mountains from its base on the east coast. In recent years the huge rescue helicopter based at Stornoway can often fly when other aircraft remain grounded but there have been times when even its take-off has had to be postponed.

The accident illustrated that there were three key players in a recurring drama: the pilots who would fly if at all possible; the local General Practitioner, who, on deciding to call for the air ambulance, had to be sure that the patient was going to benefit by evacuation; and the brave nurses from the Southern General Hospital, who volunteered to go on flights in all sorts of weather.

At the time of the accident I was doing National Service in the Royal Navy and I was travelling south from Lochmaddy on my way to join a minesweeper in the Mediterranean. On arrival at Queen Street Station, Glasgow, I was horrified to see the billboards about the crash. I had a couple of days in hand so I was able to stay in Glasgow and represent the Macleod family and the people of Uist at the funerals of Captain Calderwood and Radio Officer McGinlay. That of Sister Kennedy took place later at her home on the Isle of Coll. One of the remaining Herons was renamed in her honour and gave many years of fine service.

Problems

When the de Havilland Heron, a four-engined monoplane that could carry 20 passengers, was introduced, the Government bought two of them for British European Airways, with the arrangement that one had to be immediately available for air ambulance work but that the other could be used for the scheduled flights to the smaller islands. The aircraft was a modern and (compared with the Rapide) luxurious craft, with performance and flying capabilities far in advance of those of the old de Havilland biplanes. However the Heron had limitations on its ability to land and take off from small strips so there were a number of islands into which it could not fly.

Also available at the same time was the Scottish Aviation Twin Pioneer. This was a novel 'short take-off and landing' aircraft but it was more austere than the Heron. BEA decided against the Twin Pioneer which was unfortunate for David McIntyre and his colleagues at Prestwick who built it. Its use by BEA would have opened up many islands and it would also have been a major selling point. During the 'troubles' in Malaya the Twin Pioneer did excellent work in and out of small jungle clearings and it would have been ideal for the Scottish islands.

Loganair started to fly the Britten-Norman Islander in 1967 and it managed to serve many places that the Heron could not. The air ambulance contract changed from BEA to Loganair in 1973 and many of the BEA pilots were angry that the company had not fought harder to keep the contract by buying aircraft that would have been able to land on an expanding number of islands.

During the 'seventies the demands on the air ambulance service were increasing and on many occasions rather a long time would elapse before an aircraft would arrive. Any submissions on this to the Scottish Home and Health Department tended to be answered by a statement that 'the service was under review'. The SHHD really had no firm information on the total rise in requests for flights, as compared to actual flights performed, as the administrative system that they had asked Loganair to use was only undertaken *if* a flight was possible. Initially there was no defined record of the number of requests that could not be fulfilled. From the users' point of view there was clearly a need for a further aircraft to be available.

There were several reasons for difficulty in obtaining a flight. The arrangement of 'one for service and one for patients' was outmoded because of increased demand. Also, because of potential delay, certain doctors appeared to be placing most of their calls into the 'very urgent' category which meant that an aircraft already in the air could not be diverted even for a patient sitting at an airport over which it might be flying. Initially the Glasgow-based aircraft had to cover Orkney and Shetland and a new problem was the number of oil workers with severe alcohol problems who had to be taken by air ambulance to Aberdeen, resulting in a round trip of at least six hours.

There had also been a gradual increase in the use of the air ambulance for inter-hospital transfer of patients and organs for transplant within the United Kingdom mainland. I suggested that those inter-hospital tasks should be contracted out to another company and that the Loganair aircraft and its pilots be retained for use in the islands where special flying skills were required and where the doctor had no alternative option of treatment for his patients. Eventually that sort of system was adopted when administration of the service was taken over by the Scottish Ambulance Service.

My father, myself and Dr Macphail from Campbeltown were the only General Practitioners present at a meeting arranged by the Scottish Home and Health Department on 6th October 1976. At that meeting many constructive suggestions were put forward, but not until 1st April 1993 were these ideas incorporated into the operations plan for the new integrated service which was to be administered by the Scottish Ambulance Service and controlled from a special Air Desk at Aberdeen.

Despite the volume of work which had gone into planning, this question of requests compared to actual usage did not seem to have been studied and the new service did not include an aircraft based at Glasgow. Thankfully this was re-introduced on 15th November 1993.

With the improved resuscitation of trauma victims from island accidents, there is a need for an aircraft in which a special team can arrive, adjust the patient's management and then continue to work on the patient during the inward flight. The Super King Air B200 goes part of the way towards this but, with the Islander and the small Bölkow BO 105D helicopter at Inverness, it is still really a case of 'scoop and run'.

Helicopters

Father was continually having discussions with the pilots in relation to the service and how it could be improved. During the mid 'sixties the Heron was doing a fine job but there were numerous islands on which it could not land. The pilots told Father that helicopters and crews were now available which could give a much greater service than was currently on offer. BEA also had its own helicopter company which worked on the east coast of the UK to service the offshore oil and gas fields.

At that time there was a procedure for calling a Service helicopter by telephoning the local Medical Officer of Health and seeking his approval for the request. There was also a little booklet that was issued to each isolated General Practitioner giving him details of how to select and prepare a small landing spot for day and night use by the helicopter. There were problems with this service in that (a) the RAF's foremost commitment was to Service purposes; (b) the helicopters were based on the east coast and at times had problems flying over the mountains; (c) they required fuelling stops; and (d) the pilots had little knowledge of the west coast and the islands.

Through all the medical committees, Father fought to try to secure a helicopter service based on the west coast or in the islands. He received little support from city colleagues who filled the majority of places on the committees. However he took the fight nationwide and in 1970, when he found that the British Medical Association in Scotland had not even mentioned the problem in their annual report, he opposed the adoption of the report at the Association's Annual Representative Meeting.

At that time I was a junior member of the National Council of the BMA so I followed him to the rostrum and joined him in opposing the motion. We did not succeed but achieved favourable publicity for our effort and also created a precedent within the BMA in that it became the first occasion when a father and son had spoken in succession at the ARM.

Father continued the fight for helicopters right into his retirement and he would be delighted to know that the Scottish Ambulance Service now has a small helicopter based at Inverness and that there is a huge Coastguard helicopter based at Stornoway which has carried out numerous ambulance flights, often in very bad weather.

An Evacuation Case List

Air Ambulance use from North Uist 1985–1994

Year	1985	1986	1987	1988	1989	1990	1991	1992	1993	1994
Fixed-Wing	16	12	11	8	15	16	15	16	12	24
Helicopter	0	0	0	1	3	6	4	2	2	0
Total	16	12	11	9	18	22	19	18	14	24

The islands of North Uist and Berneray have a combined population of 1,700. There were 24 evacuations during 1994. These were all by fixed-wing aircraft as a result of the re-instatement of the Islander based at Glasgow, patients being uplifted from Benbecula Airport.

No.	Sex	Age	Diagnosis	Destination
1.	F	44	Psychiatric	Stornoway
2.	F	59	Chest	Inverness
3.	F	65	Chest	Stornoway
4.	F	85	Heart	Inverness
5.	M	70	Blocked Artery	Glasgow
6.	M	75	Acute Abdomen	Stornoway
7.	F	36	Premature Labour	Glasgow
8.	F	20	Post Operative Bleed	Glasgow
9.	F	28	Premature Labour	Glasgow
10.	M	1	Gastroenteritis	Glasgow
11.	M	85	Blocked Artery	Glasgow
12.	F	89	Broken Hip	Glasgow
13.	M	12	Appendix	Stornoway
14.	F	26	Premature Labour	Stornoway
15.	M	69	Psychiatric	Stornoway
16.	M	1	Gastroenteritis	Glasgow
17.	F	75	Acute Abdomen	Glasgow
18.	F	25	Broken Leg	Glasgow
19.	F	27	Acute Abdomen	Glasgow
20.	F	59	Chest	Inverness
21.	F	71	Heart	Inverness
22.	M	50	Meningitis	Glasgow
23.	M	86	Acute Abdomen	Glasgow
24.	F	59	Chest	Inverness

Notes

1. Nos. 2, 20 and 24 refer to the same patient.
2. Nos. 10 and 16 refer to the same patient.
3. The three pregnant patients had been booked to travel by scheduled flight at 38 weeks but each started labour early.

I have indicated earlier that the Air Ambulance Service has been of immense benefit to the people who live in the islands. This list of the patients evacuated during 1994 illustrates its value exceedingly well. All the patients required specialist medical and nursing care which was beyond the scope of local hospital services currently available.

The Ambulancemen

*T*HE TITLE of this chapter does not conform to the political correctness of the 1990s and it is used very loosely to encompass a wide range of people of both genders who made their mark on the Scottish Air Ambulance Service and whose characters have also undoubtedly been influenced by their experience with the Service. There are many whose names are not recorded here but some of those who have left an indelible mark are mentioned below.

Jimmy Orrell flew the first ambulance flight with Midland & Scottish Air Ferries, the first Scottish airline, founded by the visionary John Sword. Jimmy Orrell flew several subsequent flights and later went on to fly for Imperial Airways and BOAC. Other ambulance flights of Midland & Scottish were undertaken by Johnny Rae, Cyril Coleman and Ed Stewart. Midland & Scottish also had Winnie Drinkwater, Scotland's first female commercial pilot, on its staff and a legend in her own right.

Edmund Fresson made little record in his Flying Logs of his air ambulance flights but he is known to have undertaken many such missions and he vigorously encouraged the development of airfields in Orkney. The life-saving possibilities that they would bring were just as much in his thoughts as the planned introduction of scheduled services. Within a matter of months of Midland & Scottish Air Ferries' first flight in 1933, Fresson's Highland Airways was providing the same service in the north.

John Hankins flew for both Highland Airways and Scottish Airways, taking his experience to both the Northern Isles and the Western Isles. What became of this popular New Zealander?

Readers will already have gathered that David Barclay and the Air Ambulance Service were almost synonymous for three decades. When BEA was formed in 1947 upon the nationalisation of the private airlines, the new management, based in London, dismissed the senior management of the airlines they had taken over, with blatant contempt for their pioneering work and experience. Casualties included Edmund Fresson, George Nicholson, and David Barclay, who was Chief Pilot of Scottish Airways. However a change of heart took place in the case of Barclay when it was decided to set up an Air Ambulance Division of BEA in Scotland. In a rare display of wisdom, the BEA hierarchy realised that David Barclay was the man for the job. He dedicated the remaining 18 years of his flying career to responding to ambulance calls throughout the islands he loved so much and where he was held in high regard by many communities.

Many other pilots flew with BEA on air ambulance duties, some for short secondments to Renfrew to gain experience, others for longer periods and for them Renfrew was home. They in turn were joined by radio officers such as Hugh McGinlay and Jimmy Mitchell.

Eric Starling was Flight Manager of BEA at Glasgow from 1947 until 1968. He undertook many ambulance flights during this period and then became a full-time air ambulance captain from 1968 until retirement in 1971. Eric Starling was held in a certain awe by the pilots under his command who, when flying with David Barclay, recoiled in alarm at some of the tricks perpetuated by the latter veteran, in case news of them reached the boss's ears.

But Starling also has a mischievous sense of humour which the mantle of Flight Manager might sometimes, but not always, have inhibited. Eric Starling remains one of Scottish aviation's great characters.

Mrs A W Ferguson travelled as nurse on the very first air ambulance flight in 1933 and an island-based district nurse often carried on this tradition with subsequent flights. Margaret Boyd and Jean Govan became the first regular nurses to accompany air ambulances from Renfrew to uplift patients, a role they shared between them from 1938 until 1942. The two ladies remained close friends for many years until Jean passed away. Margaret still takes a keen interest in the development of the modern service and recalls her own contribution with nostalgia and a twinkle in her eye.

Nurses based at the Southern General Hospital in Glasgow, Balfour Hospital in Kirkwall, and Gilbert Bain Hospital in Lerwick, all established an enviable reputation with many performing a large number of missions during their off-duty hours.

The Loganair period brought its own list of notable flyers, starting with Captains Ken Foster and Duncan McIntosh. Other early names include Bill Henley, Ben Thomas, and Barney Barron. On Orkney the service was pioneered by Jim Lee and Andy Alsop; and in Shetland Alan Whitfield became a modern-day legend who has now recorded his experiences in his book, *Island Pilot*. Loganair pilots who carry on the tradition include Dave Dyer, Dave Edmondston, Malcolm Bray, and many more.

The SAS helicopter is relatively new but Captain Phil Green and his colleagues are already establishing a new folklore as they descend from the skies into the most inhospitable environments to rush people to urgent medical care. Their story is still in the making.

To list everyone who plays a part in the air ambulance service is impossible. In a single operation countless people are involved — doctors, nurses, communications personnel to co-ordinate an evacuation, pilots to fly the aircraft, engineers to ensure that aircraft are ready to take off at an instant's notice, ground staff to light up the runway of an airfield hastily opened in the middle of the night, ambulance crews summoned to provide swift and smooth road transport at both ends of the flight. Most of these people are extremely modest and will claim that they are just 'doing their job'. But they frequently go beyond the call of normal duty and every one of them has performed an heroic deed at some time or other. Just ask some of the patients whose lives have been saved by their swift action and dedication.

'That Monster'

The circumstances surrounding the second-ever air ambulance flight in Scotland are detailed in Dr John Macleod's account (on page 86). It tells how the Daily Record *newspaper was persuaded to sponsor that flight. The gesture put the newspaper in a unique position to secure a 'scoop' and its 'Special Correspondent', who signed himself merely as 'W.G.G.', was on board that historic flight to North Uist. This is how he reported the events of that journey on 22nd May 1933.*

YESTERDAY I had an adventure on behalf of the *Daily Record* in a passenger aeroplane belonging to the Midland and Scottish Ferries Ltd (sic), piloted by Captain J H Orrell, who might be described as 'Scotland's Red Cross Pilot'.

There was chartered yesterday morning an aeroplane on behalf of the Rev Malcolm Gillies, of the Clachan Church, North Uist, in the Outer Hebrides.

Mr Gillies came to Glasgow to undergo an operation some weeks ago. He is now convalescent, but such is his physical condition that it was not considered wise to take him home by the usual rail and steamer route that occupies over a day's journeying.

First Glimpse of 'Plane

The reverend gentleman wished to get back to his parish, among the people whom he tends, and it was decided to make the journey by air.

Never before had those people of the Western Islands, who have never left their native land, seen an aeroplane.

The 'plane, a Dragon Moth, carrying half-a-dozen passengers, left Renfrew Aerodrome at 11.25 a.m. We were safely landed on the white sandy beach of Baleshare Ford, North Uist, exactly 90 minutes later.

Incidentally, Captain Orrell, who was accompanied by Mr J Graham McDonald, one of the officials of the company, was doing pioneer work for Scottish aviation, and laying the foundation of a scheme advocated by the *Daily Record* about three years ago.

Historic Flight

So far as the Hebrides was concerned this flight will prove an historic one, for I understand that it is the intention of the Midland and Scottish Ferries Ltd., to link up the islands with the mainland.

The journey between Renfrew and North Uist was delightfully enjoyable. The passengers, in addition to Mr Gillies, included Mrs Gillies and Dr Macleod, in charge of the patient, and the latter thoroughly enjoyed the experience.

The route taken was by way of Oban to Ardnamurchan, the most western point of the British mainland, thence over the sea to Skye by way of the Isles of Eigg and Rhum which lay, in almost sympathetic loneliness, in a sun-kissed sea that reflected the blue of the sky.

Coolin Hills

Then, at a height of over 1,000 feet, we passed alongside, so close that we felt we could touch them, the strangely formed Cuchielean (sic), so unromantically spelt the Coolin Hills of Skye.

Down below, little more than a cairn it appeared to us, was Dunvegan Castle, the stronghold of the Macleods. Then Mr Gillies pointed to some crofts below.

'There', he said, 'is my parish, and it stretches as far as the eye can see, even from the height of the clouds which are drifting past us.'

At that point the machine nosed due west, and within ten minutes the Sea of the Hebrides had been crossed, and we were roaring over the quiet of the treeless island of North Uist.

Right to the far side we went, and 'planed gently down to a wide stretch of white sand that glittered as silver in the sunlight.

The Landing

We landed in Baleshare Ford, just a few yards from the Atlantic, and taxied for over half a mile past little lakes left by the eddying sea, and round low-lying rocks that later would be submerged by the flowing tide, until we were within a stone's throw of the manse of Clachan.

Walking along the sands was a horse and cart, tended by two young girls. The entourage stopped to gaze at us. The horse suddenly bolted. The two girls looked at one another, and apparently decided that horse sense was the better part of valour. They followed the tracks of the cart.

The 'plane of course, had been heard and seen by everyone on the island, which is 36 miles in circumference, and is the homeland of about three thousand people.

I stepped out. Between the 'plane and a little mound, on which stood a thatched house of rough grey stone, was a twenty yards' stretch of sea water, left by the ebbing tide. On the mound appeared two girls and a youth. I waved to them to come to us.

From the house stepped an old woman. She spoke to the young man. He took off his boots and stockings, and, lifting the old woman, forded the narrow stretch of water. She was Mrs McDonald, over 80 years of age, who, widowed, with two sons killed in the war, lives alone in her sheiling.

A fine old lady, and though the Gaelic is her everyday tongue, she spoke perfect English, softly intoned with the accent of the isles.

She smiled as I went to shake hands with her. 'And did *you* come out of this monster?' she asked. 'And who is with you, at all?'

When she saw the minister of her church, which is a building little bigger than her own home, she could hardly believe her eyes. I know not what was her greeting, for it was in the Gaelic.

Welcome Home

After Mrs McDonald came others, healthy tanned men of the peat fields and pretty girls of natural complexions who hid their shyness before us strangers by exchanging laughter between themselves. Maybe they made us from the city think that we were not so clever with the surprise that we had sprung on them.

And after them, the school children, who, I learned later, were given a holiday for the rest of the day.

One and all showed the greatest interest in Mrs McDonald's 'monster'. We were bombarded with questions, and Captain Orrell was the busy man answering them. They all wanted flights, but that was impossible.

We were two hours at Baleshare Ford, and in that time folk came from all parts of the island, and many of them arrived in motor-cars. One, indeed, was driven by a liveried chauffeur.

Another of the McDonalds, a youth in his teens, took our photograph, with a little box camera that contained only two unexposed films. Again that soft-spoken voice, as he handed me the film roll. 'You will send me them back?' was his injunction.

The Parting

Then for home. The starting of the powerful engines, that frightened the children, the waving of hands, the taxi-ing of the 'plane across the sands, and within a minute or so the little group was lost to our sight, as we made in the direction of Skye.

Mr Graham McDonald and I were now the only two passengers. Somehow I felt the lonely one, not like any of those islanders, who seemed to be so happy and care-free ... But I was not given time to dream much of them. Ever there was something new to catch the eye, for we came home by a more southerly route, down by Coll, over Iona, which we encircled low down several times while the islanders gazed up at us; south of Mull, across the Firth of Lorne and Loch Fyne, roaring over pretty Lochgilphead and gloomy-looking Loch Striven, to the Clyde. Easy home then.

(This article appeared in the Daily Record of 23rd May 1933 and is reproduced by kind permission of the Editor.)

Where Dragons Dare

*E*SHA NESS, at the extreme northwestern corner of the Shetland mainland, 40 miles from Lerwick, is served by a meandering and undulating road which is, even today, a severe test of driving competence. No aircraft had ever landed at Esha Ness before 30th April 1937, and none is likely to have landed there ever since.

On that date the circumstances were exceptional. Alex MacRae, the 51-year-old lighthouse keeper who diligently warned ships of the rocks and cliffs surrounding this Shetland promontory, had taken seriously ill. Two doctors had tended Mr MacRae and both agreed that he had to be airlifted urgently for emergency hospital treatment.

The doctors telegraphed the Edinburgh headquarters of the Northern Lighthouse Board to advise them of the situation and that to move the keeper by road to hospital in Lerwick would be far too dangerous. The Board got in touch with Allied Airways of Aberdeen which informed it that an aircraft could be despatched to Sumburgh airfield, at the extreme southern tip of the Mainland.

But that would not solve the problem. The patient would still have to be taken on the tortuous road journey to Lerwick, and then a further 25 miles to reach the airfield. Could the aircraft land at Esha Ness?

The man who was charged with the task of trying was Captain Henry Vallance. At 7.30am he set off from his operational base at Thurso in one of Allied's de Havilland Dragons.

'When I reached Esha Ness', recalled Vallance, 'there was mist blanketing the lighthouse making visibility very poor. I circled for a time until the sun dispersed the mist sufficiently for me to attempt a dummy landing. The keeper's son and daughter were awaiting my arrival. They had cleared a small landing area but it was extremely dangerous as I had to pass over an inlet which had dug a deep chasm in the cliffs below the lighthouse. An updraft funnelling through this gaping cleft in the rocks could have had a serious effect on the lightly built seven-passenger aircraft.'

'However on the second approach to the cleared area of land I was able to put the aircraft down. The aircraft's seats had been removed at Thurso and Mr MacRae was carried from the lighthouse 200 yards away and placed on a mattress inside the cabin.'

'Taking off was even more difficult than the landing. The patch that had been cleared was inadequate for the aircraft to take a proper run before reaching an area of uncleared stony ground. The ground sloped downwards and there was no breeze which would have been a welcome asset. I pulled the aircraft upwards and it did leave the ground but in reality it was continuing horizontally and not gaining altitude. It was the sloping ground that was leaving the aircraft, not the other way around.'

'The de Havilland Dragon was an extremely manoeuvrable aircraft that could operate from the smallest of fields. Several other aircraft types could have landed successfully at Esha Ness. But I don't think there are many of them that could have taken off again.'

Having become airborne once more, Henry Vallance proceeded southwards to Edinburgh, calling at Thurso en route to refuel. It was a journey that took approximately five hours.

'I never knew the cause of Mr MacRae's illness', Vallance recollected, 54 years after the event. 'Charlotte MacRae, the patient's wife, and Nurse McVey travelled with him but they were both in the back of the aircraft and I had little contact with them. I was only twenty-one at the time and would have been nervous about enquiring. Maybe they wouldn't have told me anyway. The sad thing is that having reached the hospital safely, Mr MacRae died a week later.'

Henry Vallance flew with Scottish Airways during the Second World War when the airline struggled to keep a skeleton air service operational to counter the isolation that its absence would have brought to the islands.

'I don't recall undertaking any ambulance flights during this period', reflected Vallance, 'but early in the war I flew in search of a missing merchant ship up and down the Hebrides. Then there was a tragic incident off Liverpool when men were trapped inside a capsized submarine that protruded vertically from the water. The most experienced divers were to be found working on the scuttled German First World War fleet in Scapa Flow and I had the job of rushing a diving team down to Liverpool.'

Captain Vallance never had reason to fly in the vicinity of Esha Ness during the rest of his time flying the Scottish air routes. After the Second World War he was a Captain with KLM Royal Dutch Airlines. 'One of my routes with KLM was from Amsterdam to Tokyo via Anchorage. The flightpath regularly passed over Shetland. I would be at a height in excess of 30,000 feet but there were occasions when I could just pick out a small dot that was Esha Ness Lighthouse.'

The aircraft then under his command was the Douglas DC-8 which certainly could not have emulated the feat performed by the frail Dragon in 1937. The DC-8's wingspan was almost as long as the Dragon's take-off run.

Two Pioneer Nurses

*M*ARGARET BOYD, in her 88th year, gazed in awe at the array of life-saving equipment on board the Bölkow helicopters at the launch of the re-organised air ambulance service at Prestwick Airport on 26th March 1993. The occasion marked 55 years since Margaret had flown as the first regular air ambulance nurse from Renfrew to Islay on 4th March 1938.

'In 1938 everything was very primitive. We landed on fields that had no marked runway and the flares to direct the pilot on island airstrips consisted of pails arranged in two parallel rows and containing paraffin rags. These were lit to indicate the direction of the wind and the area of the field in which he should land.'

'For my first flight I was given a flight ticket. It consisted of a piece of paper which showed just my name and my destination.'

'One of my first flights was for a young man by the name of Angus MacVicar. He was very ill indeed and Coats of Paisley arranged a private charter to bring him to Dr Crockett's clinic. He had a chest condition which later on turned out to be brucellosis. He had a remarkable recovery.'

'My only equipment was a first aid box in a small case. On one occasion at Campbeltown the aeroplane would not start and a phone call had to be made for a second aircraft. We had to wait for about an hour-and-a-half. My patient had a perforated ulcer and his condition appeared to be getting worse. I called the doctor and he gave the patient an injection of morphine to settle him down. We eventually arrived at Glasgow.'

'Our crew consisted of my friend Miss Jean Govan, Captain David Barclay and Wireless Operator Hugh Black. The four of us were the main crew for a long time. At Renfrew our waiting place was a small hut with just a central stove and there we drank many cups of tea while we were waiting. Upon almost every occasion we were in the air within ten minutes of having the telephone call.'

'The airport staff would phone Mr Lochhead who had a garage in Greenock Road, Paisley, and they phoned us at the same time. Mr Lochhead quickly arrived to pick us up and when we arrived at Renfrew Aerodrome the plane was ticking over in readiness.'

'Captain Barclay seemed to be just perfect in his workmanship because he could land anywhere. Most of the landings took place on bare fields. Sometimes sheep had to be cleared to give us room. Other times we landed on the beach with the ground very soft and if we had to wait a long time for the patient the plane kept sinking into the sand. The patient didn't leave the house until the plane had safely landed so we usually had some time to wait while he was carried over the fields on a stretcher.'

'On one occasion during the summer, Captain Barclay's family were on holiday at Rothesay and he dipped down very low in the bay so that his two daughters and wife could wave to him. I think that the children would have been delighted.' (Captain Barclay's daughter, Sheila, recalls that her father regularly did this when they were holidaying at Rothesay and Millport. He also used to fly low over their house in Bishopton so that their mother knew to expect him home — until a neighbour registered a complaint.)

'One time during the war I was coming in from Barra on a beautiful summer's day when I saw a shadow in the water. It had the appearance of a submarine so I thought I had better go forward and let Captain Barclay and the navigator know what I had seen. They burst out laughing because they immediately realised that it was just the shadow of our plane on the water.'

'Another time I had an all-night flight. We set off at 00.20am to Islay in very bad weather, atrocious. You could see nothing but the rain splashing down on the windows. I was sitting in the back of the fuselage. It was a very old-fashioned plane, the Spartan Cruiser, and the pilot and navigator were boxed-off in the cockpit.'

'As a rule we would take three-quarters of an hour in day-time to reach Islay, so I thought it must take much longer at night. But having left shortly after midnight, I looked at my watch and we were still in the air at 2.00am. I thought that there must be something strange so I took out my ticket to make sure it was Islay I was going to. Sure enough, it said Islay. All I could do was sit and wait.'

'After a long time, through the rainy windows I could see a red lighthouse. I was sure that there was no red lighthouse near Islay. We landed eventually at 3.00am. on Islay. I asked Captain Barclay about the red lighthouse. ''Oh'', he said, ''We were off the north coast of Ireland. The navigator was getting messages from Renfrew Airport and Newtownards Airport in Ireland causing a mix-up until we flew north to Islay.''

'As previously mentioned, the patient did not leave the house until the plane had safely landed. The patient, an elderly lady whose husband was very bad with arthritis, had some distance to come. She was travelling to Glasgow Royal Infirmary for an abdominal operation. Captain Barclay had decided that he would return over Arran, but to do so he had to fly higher than usual and, being winter time, it was a bit risky. Little did I know how risky, until he told me three months later.'

'While flying so high, the plane's wings had frozen, an engine had stalled and I had a funny sensation of being suctioned back to my seat. I could not move, my hands swelled, my brain and my feet — it was a queer sensation. I thought I would get up and see how my patient was but I was once again suctioned to the back of my seat and there I had to wait. It all happened within a short time. Just seconds, but it happened twice.'

'When I got back to the airport at Renfrew, I said to Captain Barclay, "What kind of sensation was that we had tonight?" and he said, "Oh, just weather conditions." However three months later he told me that the wings had frozen, an engine had stopped and we had gone into a nose-dive. He managed to level the aircraft out and restart the engine, but no sooner had it started again and the same thing happened. This time we were much lower in height and he said to Hugh Black, "This is it, this time. We've had it."

'Just at that moment he noticed the Greenock lights and with all his strength he managed to level the aircraft again. The engine and wings defrosted and we got home safely. From that moment on I began to realise what a risk there was with each journey. Thereafter I always had a quiet prayer for a safe return whenever I went flying.' *

'Another experience of consequence occurred during the day. I was called out three times in the one day. The flight started at 5.30am with a glorious sunrise making the earth into a great big orange ball with the sun in the horizon. When we returned from the first journey we were told of the second, and the same with the third with only space for some black tarry tea in between.'

'I took turn about with each flight with my friend Jean Govan. I had a lot of difficulty at first coaxing Jean to take it on until eventually she agreed that we do it.'

'On one occasion Jean had to go to Benbecula but when they arrived it was too foggy to land. They continued to Barra and when they got out the pilot said, "Well, here we are nurse. We'll have to stay the night on Barra." "Oh no," says she, "I can't. I must get back." But he said, "I can't go back. So neither can you." She was reconciled to the situation and the three of them stayed in a hotel. That was the day that Neville Chamberlain's efforts to conclude a peace agreement with Adolf Hitler following Germany's invasion of Poland ended in failure. Before Jean got back the next day, we were at war.'

'Some months later this young pilot met Jean and he said to her, in the small room where we gathered for our cups of tea, with a number of pilots around the fire, "Hello nurse. I haven't seen you since the night we spent in the hotel on Barra." Jean felt very embarrassed.'

'Jean's most memorable call-out was to South Uist for an expectant mother to come to Rottenrow Hospital. As a rule, we were told, there would be no midwifery cases but this was a real emergency. The aircraft arrived at Askernish and the expectant mother was put aboard with her husband accompanying her. Before she went on the plane, the doctor explained to Jean that the patient was expecting twins and there were complications. He gave Jean morphine for administering during the flight.'

'Captain Barclay flew as high as he could, thinking this might help a bit. However over the Minch the mother was in labour and her husband was ushered into the front of the cabin. The babies, Siamese twins, were stillborn. The mother wanted to turn back for home but Jean explained that she had to go to hospital. When she arrived at Renfrew Airport, most unexpectedly, reporters were waiting.'

'The following day reporters insisted on hanging around at our door. For three days this continued. Then on the third day there was a pit disaster in Wales and that was the only reason that they finally left. Jean would not give any account of the case nor would she be photographed.' **

'A month later Dr Shearer visited, in the company of an official, to ask Jean if she would accept the OBE. Her first question was, "Can two of us have it?" "No, it is only for one." So Jean refused, saying, "We are both doing the same work."'

'During the war the pilot had to set off "fairy lights" upon our return to Renfrew before he got permission to land. The war also curtailed the involvement of our Association because we only employed trained nurses and they were soon being called up for war service. With our numbers depleted, we turned the big house that we used into a nursing home which mainly handled midwifery cases. But with a reduced staff we had to give up the air ambulance flying. From this point in 1942 the Southern General Hospital in Glasgow provided volunteer nurses for the service.'

* This flight took place on 27th March 1938 with Spartan Cruiser G-ACSM. The patient was 73-year-old Mrs Mary Bell of Bowmore. She died shortly after admission to Glasgow's Western Infirmary. G-ACSM was requisitioned by the RAF on 2nd April 1940.

** The Siamese twins were stillborn over the Isle of Mull on de Havilland DH84 Dragon G-ACNG on 9th May 1938.

Poetic Pigs and Piccadilly Highlanders

This article by A L Lloyd appeared in the magazine Picture Post *of 14th June 1947, only a few months after BEA took over the responsibility for the Scottish Air Ambulance Service. It comes via Wendy Johnson whose late husband, Captain Bill Johnson, was seconded from the RAF in 1942 to assist with civil flying, and he featured in the photographs which accompanied the article.*

*T*IME, TO the distress of many, marches on. In the Hebrides, once so wild and remote, the girls sing *Open the Door, Richard* and the boys follow Dick Barton. Even on the grey mist-shrouded island of Barra — a place which Samuel Johnson considered too outlandish to visit on his celebrated tour — there are four film shows a week. Out in the sea is Ciosmaol Castle, the old pirate stronghold of The MacNeils of Barra. Over it, the twice-a-day plane flies with the Late Extra papers.

Townfolk and trippers regret all this. What they want from the Western Islands (just for a fortnight, anyway), is something austere and fey and primitive; some kind of life to match the glistening grey rocks and the peat-smoke and the potatoes laid out in their queer grave-like lazy-beds on the hillside. People who don't have to live there would prefer the Islands to be the backward old backwaters they once were, when folk crouched in smoky hovels with turf-and-bracken roofs, and lived off a diet of cockles and potatoes and strong stewed tea, and encountered ghosts and fairies at every twist and turn. The islanders know better. They see no reason why they should live like fine poetic pigs just to please a bunch of visitors in shop-bought kilts (Piccadilly Highlanders, they call them; to the Islander, the sight of a kilt is comical or embarrassing).

Civilisation, with all its benefits and many of its banes as well, has come fast to the Islands. And if you ask what has been the biggest single step forward over the last decade or so, the Hebridean will probably plump for the air ambulance service. Men were tough in the old days (they are now), but illness was a terror all the time on the Islands. Water from the surface wells spread epidemics of typhus; the old habit of passing the pipe around (a man was stingy if he didn't) encouraged the most malignant kinds of consumption. Appendicitis was fatal. To break a leg meant generally becoming a cripple.

Till fifty years ago, there was no doctor on islands like Barra. Even today, hospitals are scarce (there is a good one in Stornoway, a small one on the Campbeltown peninsula, and a fever hospital on Islay — that is all). Until twelve years ago, any islander meeting with an accident, or falling suddenly ill, might have to wait two or three days for the steamer to call, and then make a hard two-day journey by sea, rail, and road, before reaching hospital in Glasgow or Edinburgh. Nowadays, with the air service, the whole trip can be done in three or four hours. In their twelve years of operation, the ambulance craft have averaged two or three calls a week, and have carried well over a thousand patients.

The air ambulance service is run nowadays by the Scottish Division of British European Airways, who operate a regular line of DH Rapide biplanes to the Western Islands for carrying passengers and freight. If one of the doctors of the Highlands and Islands Medical Service has a patient in urgent need of transport, they take the seats out of one of the regular planes, and put in a stretcher instead. One of the big Glasgow hospitals, the Southern General, has a rota of volunteer nurses always on call for the air ambulance; and as a rule, within half-an-hour of receiving the call from the island, the plane is leaving Renfrew airport on its hundred-mile-or-so trip across the rocks and lochs and over the wild seas that race up the Gulf of the Hebrides.

The trip, though short, is no picnic. The weather is treacherous and quick-changing. Before the war, too, patients had often to be picked up from mere fields, and landing was a nightmare. During the war, however, the islands were used by the RAF guarding the Western Approaches, and most of them have well-built airstrips which the civil planes can use. Some of the islands — Barra, for instance — have imposing stretches of flat cockle strand which make a fine firm landing-ground almost as soon as the tide has gone.

The ambulance journey costs £12 10s an hour (that is about £40 for the round trip). Even for folk who can make £3 a night in good times at lobster-fishing, that's a lot of money. The fare is paid, as a rule, by the County Councils of Argyll and Inverness-shire, who look after the Hebrides between them.

Typical of scores of cases was the affair of the lighthouse-keeper's daughter on the Monach Isles, west of the Outer Hebrides. There the doctor had arranged to signal to the ambulance pilot with a white sheet, if the case was urgent. The plane put out over the Atlantic on spec, the white signal was spotted; and after cruising round the jagged sea-rocks for a while, the pilot touched down on the tiny island of Heisker, a mile-and-a-half from the lighthouse island. The sick girl was rowed across the sound, and the aircraft contrived to take off again. The girl reached the hospital in the nick of time. *

Those who think the aeroplane age has spoilt the Hebridean's simple life should try talking to one of those same islanders. He would be able to tell them a thing or two that might cause them to change their minds, especially if they got him chatting about the planes of the Air Ambulance Service.

* The Monach Isles, to the west of North Uist, are also known as the Heiskers. The two larger islands in the group are Ceann Iar and Ceann Ear. To the west of Ceann Iar is Shillay, a small island on which the lighthouse is situated. On 26th April 1937 news that Lighthouse-keeper McKenzie's 17-year-old daughter was ill with appendicitis was transmitted by radio to the airfield at Sollas. Dr Alex Macleod from Lochmaddy had reached Shillay after great difficulty on the previous night and he said that, if the pilot would pass over the island, he would wave a white handkerchief if help was needed. When Captain John Hankins flew low over the lighthouse he saw the white handkerchief fluttering in the wind. There was no possibility of a landing on Shillay but he managed to alight at Hearnish at the northern tip of Ceann Iar, no mean feat in the large three-engined Spartan Cruiser. Betty McKenzie and the doctor were taken by open boat across the Sound of Shillay and put on board the plane. Hankins then proceeded to Barra to pick up another ambulance case, 18-year-old Mary McDougall, and three other passengers, one of whom was the novelist Compton McKenzie, before continuing to Renfrew. This event is recalled by Dr J A J Macleod in Chapter 8 — it was his father, Dr Alex J Macleod who featured in the Shillay lighthouse event.

Alick Macaulay of Paiblesgarry, fills in some background to the Monach Islands at that time. 'I was once told by a pupil at the island school that a plane had landed on Monach before the war. This one landed on Ceann Ear and the teacher took the class to see the plane. He was actually allowed inside the aircraft which he describes as very small with a large propeller. The landing area, if in grass at the time, was quite spacious and capable of small plane landings. It is also possible to land on Ceann Iar above Cròic Bay, which is much nearer Shillay and its lighthouse. On 15th November 1936 two light keepers, James Milne and Ward Black, were drowned on the Sound of Shillay on their way back from Ceann Iar. During this period only two families lived on Monach, both Macdonald. The islands were evacuated in 1942 by them.'

The Trawlerman's Son

The name of David Barclay is synonymous with the development of aviation in the Western Isles and with the Scottish Air Ambulance Service. He flew his first ambulance flight on 27th May 1935 with Northern and Scottish Airways Ltd and when he flew his last ambulance mission on 29th April 1965 he had flown more than 1,200 ambulance flights. Captain Barclay recorded some of his experiences shortly after his retiral.

PEERING INTO the night from the storm-lashed cockpit of the Rapide, all I could see were my navigation lights. From the dark void ahead, above, and below, the weather

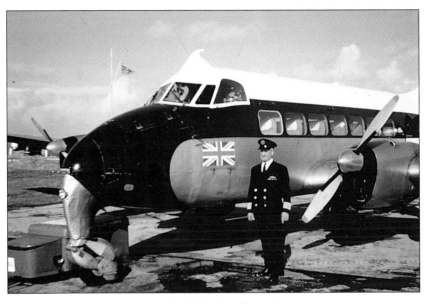

Captain David Barclay at Tiree, 1962.
(Photo by Captain Keith Warburton)

David Barclay at the controls of the Heron, 1962.
(Photo by Captain Keith Warburton)

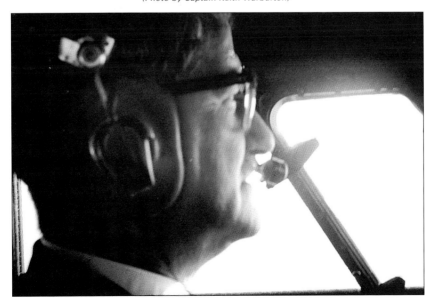

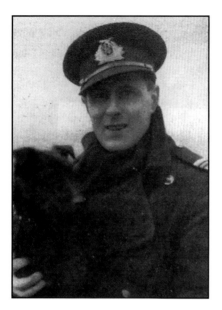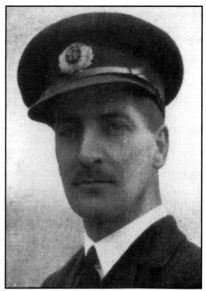

Northern & Scottish Airways' Captain John Hankins and Captain David Barclay
(Photo courtesy of Bill Palmer)

Margaret Boyd, the first regular air ambulance nurse.
(Photo courtesy of Margaret Boyd)

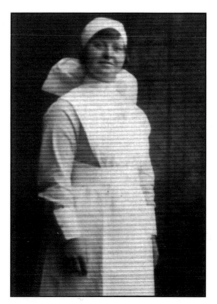

Shetland

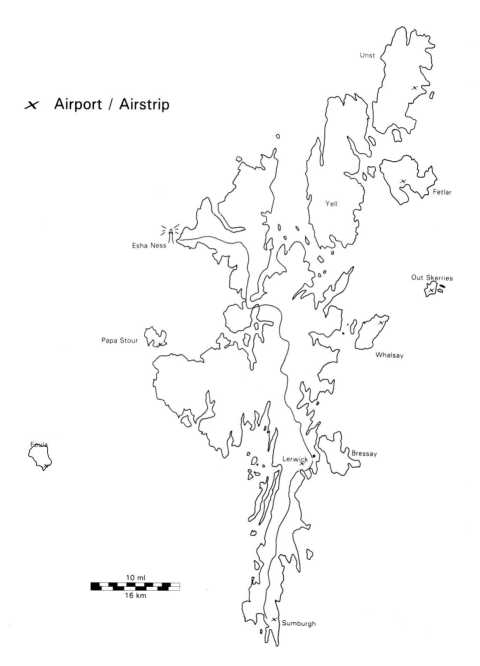

✗ Airport / Airstrip

Unst

Fetlar

Yell

Esha Ness

Out Skerries

Papa Stour

Whalsay

Foula

Bressay

Lerwick

10 ml
16 km

Sumburgh

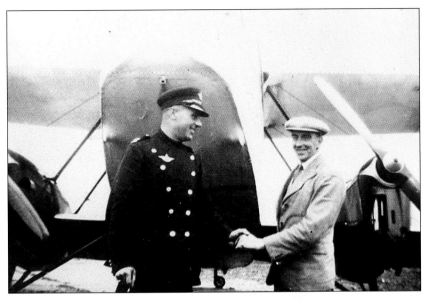

James McGeachy *(right)* with the pilot of a Midland & Scottish
Air Ferries Dragon at Campbeltown in 1934.
(Photo courtesy of Captain Ken Foster)

Captain Henry Vallance reminisces over an illustrious flying career.
(Photo Island Photographic Co. Ltd., Douglas, Isle of Man)

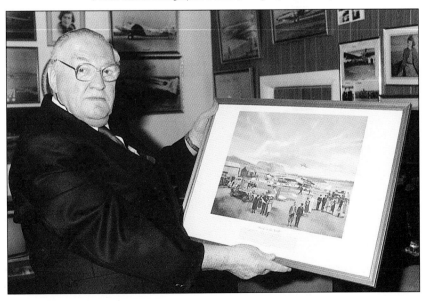

seemed to be hurling everything at the light aircraft to stop me from keeping an urgent appointment on lonely Benbecula island.

I was flying blind but, in my mind's eye I could see the scene in the wild Atlantic rollers about a mile below, where a tiny trawler was battling its way to port. I reckoned the skipper wouldn't be making more than eight knots in the dreadful conditions. He had a critically ill boy of eleven on board and each minute would seem like an hour.

Every second was vital in the youngster's fight for survival. He had peritonitis and his only hope lay in reaching a Glasgow hospital within the next two or three hours.

Only the air ambulance service could save his life. This was why I had taken off from Renfrew in the teeth of a storm around ten o'clock on a bitter October's night.

I had been given a brief outline of the case. The teenage patient was the son of the chief engineer on a Milford Haven trawler. On holiday, he had persuaded his father to take him on a trip to the fishing grounds.

On the way the boy had taken ill and, at first, was thought to be suffering from sea-sickness. But when his condition worsened his father realised it was something more serious. It was decided to put into Castlebay, Barra, to get him to a doctor.

Almost immediately the G.P. came up with a diagnosis — peritonitis. Then he telephoned Renfrew to ask for an air ambulance flight right away, making it quite clear his request carried a top priority classification. There was one big snag. The only airfield with night-landing facilities was at Benbecula, over 40 miles away.

Before the trawler headed out into the Atlantic once more the doctor got hold of all the penicillin he could get on the island and pumped it into the boy.

The mercy dash fell into three distinct phases. A sea passage of about 20 miles from Castlebay to Lochboisdale, a road ambulance journey — again more than 20 miles — from there to Benbecula airstrip and, finally, a flight to Glasgow.

It was getting on for midnight as I began my descent, keyed up for my first glimpse of landing lights. Down through the cloud I dropped, an anxious eye on the altimeter. Suddenly, there they were, leaping up at me from the darkness, and the tension eased a little as I swept in to land. So far, so good.

But there was no sign of the ambulance. One of the ground staff told me it hadn't arrived. I spent an hour worrying about my patient, and my aircraft, which was in danger of being blown over by the gusting wind. As a precaution I recruited four stalwart islanders and stationed two at each wing tip. When the gale reached its fiercest they used their full weight to make sure the Rapide stayed on the ground.

At last the ambulance roared into the airfield and drew up alongside the plane. Carefully, the boy was lifted out on a stretcher and made as comfortable as possible in the plane by the nurse who had flown up with me. He really was in a bad way, and I lost no time in getting airborne.

Barely one-and-three-quarter hours later I was taxi-ing to a halt at Renfrew, where a waiting ambulance rushed the youngster to hospital. That was my part of the operation over. But I just couldn't relax until I knew whether or not our efforts had been in vain.

I called the hospital every day and for the first week the boy was delirious and dangerously ill. Then, after a fortnight, he began to pick up and I was assured he would make a full recovery.

An exceptionally busy spell followed for the air ambulance service and, when I next contacted the hospital to check on the boy's progress, I was told he had been allowed home a few days before. I was delighted in one way by this news, but sorry I hadn't been able to have a word with him before he was discharged.

Four years later, in a radio broadcast, I mentioned this case and my regret at losing track of the teenager. Less than a week later a letter reached my home from his mother, who had heard the programme. Along with it came a photograph of her son, showing a strapping laddie of about 15 — a really healthy looking specimen. She thanked me for helping to save his life.

Extracted from an article which appeared in the Courier & Advertiser *of Dundee in 1968 and reproduced by kind permission of the Editor and of Mrs Sheila Harper (née Barclay). The flight described took place on 17th October 1949 with Captain Barclay at the controls of BEA de Havilland Rapide G-AHXZ.*

Rapide Response

The introduction of the National Health Service (NHS) in 1948 put the Scottish Air Ambulance Service on to a much sounder footing. But the days of a service providing round-the-clock cover 365 days of the year were still some time off. And stringent rules regulating pilots' flying hours had yet to be introduced. The name of the author of the following night call-out scenario during that period is not recorded but the events related give the full flavour of how the regularised service operated during the early NHS years.

N IGHT AMBULANCE trips are usually made by pilots and crews during their off-duty time and with the co-operation of the ground staffs. These men may be hauled from their firesides or beds to return to the aerodrome for a further spell of duty which may keep them up all night. And if the call should come from the Hebrides, ground staffs at Benbecula and Tiree have to be enlisted — no easy matter in islands where there are but few telephones and the men are scattered in farmhouses and cottages.

Just what happens when a call comes for an ambulance at night? Let us take a comparatively simple one — a call from Campbeltown at nine o'clock at night. It is James MacGeachy, the BEA official in charge, on the phone. The case is urgent. A life is at stake. The only hope is to get the patient to hospital in a few hours. This time it is a child. James has already had a frantic time rallying the ground crews, ferreting them from their corners in different parts of the countryside. He knows it is useless to phone Renfrew unless he has mustered his forces at Campbeltown. James is a native of the district and the misfortunes of his neighbours quite rightly arouse his staunchest efforts. The Station Superintendent at Renfrew promises to ring back if arrangements can be made.

In the next few minutes the switchboard at Renfrew is busy. A call to the Met Office for a weather forecast. Can a late radio watch be kept? Yes. A Rapide to be got ready for immediate take-off; full tanks as the load will be light. Ground crews and fire pickets ordered to remain on duty. A nurse for the trip from the Southern General Hospital.

Then the pilot. That's another problem. And the wireless operator, but let's not think about that yet. The standby pilot covering the period of the scheduled services has gone home and he lives too far away to be recalled. There is a pilot on the ambulance roster whose house is near the aerodrome, but he has been called out a lot lately, and anyway, he has done a hard day's airline flying. Perhaps Captain . . . will take it. He is due to land in a few minutes on the late Belfast service. The weather doesn't look too good but he will have a better idea of it than anybody as he has been very near Campbeltown on his way in. Now the decision rests with him. We can scarcely blame him if he refuses. He has an hour's motor journey to get home after he has finished flying. (We might mention at this point that, owing to housing difficulties, many of the pilots and crew live a considerable distance from the airport, some as far as the coast.)

He lands. We put up the proposition. He decides to go. A child? He has children of his own. Inwardly he is thinking that he doesn't care much for this trip in a Rapide. The Dakota trip hadn't been too easy and the Rapide hadn't half the night flying equipment.

Everything is set, nurse and wireless operator on board, stretcher in place. They take off. The pilot decides to fly direct over the Arran mountains as the clouds are clear of ice below 5,000 feet. It is thick cloud the whole way and all he sees outside is the glow of his wingtip lights reflected off the mist. After twenty-five minutes flying he reckons he is within five minutes of his destination, but his wireless operator cannot raise Campbeltown. Has there been a hitch in the arrangements? He consoles himself with the thought that it takes him as long to fly from Renfrew to Campbeltown as it takes the ground crews to get from their homes to the aerodrome. Then sure and strong comes a reply to his calls. Visibility three miles, clouds eight hundred feet — does he want a procedure let down? He does and wireless bearings at the rate of six a minute start coming in. So does the rain and his trouser legs are soaking wet. The reflection of his dashboard lights in the windscreen almost dazzle him. No modern cockpit lighting in this aircraft. He suddenly realises the lights he sees are not reflections but the real and welcome lights of the airport ahead of him. A friendly green light is flashed and he makes a better landing than he expected.

Little time is wasted in putting the child aboard with his mother, who has decided to accompany him.

All goes well on the return trip but he is sent up to 5,000 feet in order to avoid a Skymaster outward bound from Prestwick to Iceland. This takes him above the clouds but the sight of the moon gives him small satisfaction. There is all the mirk below in the Clyde estuary and he hopes it has not come too close to the ground at Renfrew. His luck is in and, after another string of bearings, he finds himself in a good position for landing when he breaks cloud.

The time is eleven thirty. He and his crew are very tired. So are dozens of ground crew who made the trip possible, but they do not complain. Their work for the Ambulance Service is, in a sense, a mission, not to be measured in hours of duty.

MacGeachy of Campbeltown

*I*N THE 1933 brochure of Midland & Scottish Air Ferries, an introduction to the section headed 'Types of Planes Available' reads: *It would perhaps be appropriate here to begin with the Company's latest acquisition — The Flying Hospital. The first of its kind in Scotland it will be used to convey serious cases from the Highlands and Islands to any Infirmary or Hospital in Glasgow. The benefits of such a service are manifest. Patients requiring skilled medical attention can receive the treatment they need within an hour of the airport's notification on request. Provision can be made for the patient receiving attention during the flight, an important and thoughtful point. Special rates, it should be mentioned, are available for urgent cases requiring ambulance machines.*

One family became associated with Midland & Scottish during the earliest days of the company, and continued to serve the needs of airlines and passengers as the names on the aircraft changed successively to Northern & Scottish Airways, Scottish Airways, and British European Airways. This was the MacGeachy family of Campbeltown where for many years James MacGeachy was the local airline representative. For his daughter Catherine, aircraft were as much part of every day living as dolls might be to her childhood friends.

'In a way I grew up with the service and my years spent at home were centred around air travel. In the early days, my father sent in weather reports to the Meteorological Office. A phone call booked at one minute to each hour came from the Met Office and we could be walking down the Main Street and the next thing we would be rushing into the nearest shop to accept the call at that number. It was coded and consisted of groups of numbers. If it was impossible for my father to take the call for some reason, my mother was left in charge of the message with strict instructions to alter it accordingly if this or that happened.'

'An old Bakelite wireless was used to give wind direction. A weather vane, in the shape of a model plane, protruded from our roof and led to the set in the bedroom, which lit up with various torchlight bulbs to give wind readings, while we were still in bed. This helped greatly with the Air Ambulance Service when on-the-spot weather reports could be given.'

'In the years when I worked with my father (1945-1954), on the Air Ambulance side the team work was marvellous. The aim was to arrive with the patients when the aircraft was landing. Most of the patients were collected from their homes and, as soon as the aircraft was airborne from Renfrew, the patient was then collected. By the time it took to get to the airfield at Machrihanish, about thirty minutes, the aircraft was touching down. So there was hardly any delay and the turn-round just took minutes.'

'On occasion, if a maternity case was unable to travel, a gynaecologist and an assistant would come down by Air Ambulance to the patient. The aircraft would normally stand by to take the gynaecologists back to Renfrew.'

Gordon MacGeachy, grandson of James MacGeachy and now a resident of Racine, Wisconsin, was intrigued when he picked up an American magazine in 1987, to find that the old man's aura lives on. In an article which covered bygone travel across the world, the writer also remembered Campbeltown. 'Airline reservation systems in the early Fifties were often quite primitive — and light-years away from today's computerized centers. In BEA's Glasgow space-control office, where I worked, each booking was handwritten, gummed down on a master control card and filed away. But nothing was quite as informal as the system used by the officer in charge in the coastal town of Campbeltown, which was served by the venerable Douglas DC-3s, the utilitarian wartime transports that were converted to civilian duty.'

'The would-be passenger would stop our man on the main street of Campbeltown to ask if he had a seat to Glasgow. They would step into the nearest door-way, out of the usual wind and rain. Then, doffing his BEA uniform cap, the official would pull out a booking card and jot down the reservation before both of them continued on their merry way.'

The writer, David Gollan, had worked for BEA in Glasgow before migrating to the USA in 1956. He confirmed that, 'Jimmy was a beloved character, one of several in the Scottish division, and kept the bookings literally "in his head." Before David Gollan had made his trans-Atlantic migration, another writer was using James MacGeachy as an introduction to an article on Scottish aviation in the *The Geographical Magazine* of October 1954.

'Romance, in the normal run of things, is not conspicuous in the hardware trade. But twenty-one years ago, enchantment, in a particularly lasting form, hit Mr James MacGeachy, ironmonger of Campbeltown in the county of Argyll. This happened one day in 1933 when a character called John Sword, a one-time baker who had made a fortune running buses in the Glasgow district, decided to spread his wings and open an air service between Renfrew (Glasgow's nearest airport) and Campbeltown and Islay.'

'This venture worked rather like a cyclotron on James MacGeachy. It split his business personality and changed the pattern of his life. He took air transport under his wing and gave it a citadel in his shop. He became the first representative of an airline in Scotland. His daughter, Catherine, was the first babe in arms to fly by a Scottish commercial air service. Today she wears the uniform of British European Airways in Campbeltown.'

'So does her papa. He represents BEA's local interests. But "local interests" is really a beggarly phrase. James MacGeachy's mind ranges far beyond the prized but limited attractions of a thirty-minute flight instead of an eight-hour sail from Glasgow to Campbeltown. He thinks in terms of continents and oceans, and in his shop he keeps a map which shows in detail the airline connections between Campbeltown and the farthest corners of the earth. He is a man who has seen some very far-fetched dreams come true.'

Time for Tea at Sollas

The hospitality offered by Dr Macleod of North Uist has gone down in Scottish aviation folklore along with the exploits of the crews who flew ambulance aircraft to North Uist and Benbecula. Captain David Barclay was undoubtedly one of the greatest beneficiaries of the Macleod 'treatment'.

*T*HE DOCTOR'S instructions seemed simple enough as I prepared for take-off. 'Make it as fast as you can and don't go above 1,000 feet because the patient has severe head injuries and the slightest pressure could be fatal.'

But there were two big snags. I had flown out to Sollas, North Uist, to answer Dr Macleod's ambulance call in early evening, and it was now almost dark. And the fastest route involved flying over mountains much higher than 1,000 feet.

This was going to be one of the few occasions when the long way round, keeping over the sea as much as possible, would be safest. And at a height of around 500 feet, I would be able to navigate from the powerful beams of the many lighthouses necessary as shipping aids throughout the treacherous waters of the west coast.

Fortunately it was a lovely clear night with a high cloud base — around 1,500 feet. The patient's critical condition meant the normal 150-mile flight from Sollas to Renfrew would be stretched out to over 200. (A long way at a pretty constant 500 feet above the inky sea.)

As I climbed gently to my self-imposed shallow ceiling I realised I was going to need every ounce of concentration to conclude this flight successfully. My first bearing came from Usinish light, on the north-east corner of South Uist. Not long afterwards I picked up the sweeping beam of Òigh-sgeir, south of the Isle of Canna.

Next landmark was Skerryvore, from which I took a line on our airstrip at Tiree, over which I flew. Then, dead ahead, west of Colonsay, the beacon of Dubh Artach gave me another 'fix'.

Over Portnahaven light, on the south-west tip of Islay, I came round in a gentle left-hand turn, following the beams of Machrihanish, Davaar and Pladda to cross the mainland at Ardrossan.

The last lap took me up the Lochwinnoch valley to Renfrew. By the time I landed I was limp but jubilant. I had done the 230-mile trip in the dark without once being over 1,000 feet.

On another memorable day I logged 7 hours 43 minutes flying time answering ambulance calls which took me almost right round Scotland.

My shift began about 9.45am with an S.O.S. from Benbecula to collect a patient who had to be taken to Stornoway Hospital in a hurry. When I touched down at Stornoway I found they were waiting for me to rush a patient to Aberdeen. We landed there at tea-time, saw the patient safely on his way, then headed for a quick cup of tea and a bite to eat.

We had hardly started when 'Ops', Renfrew, came on the phone. 'Sorry to trouble you', said the controller, 'but we have an urgent request for an ambulance to pick up a patient from Sollas, North Uist, and bring him to Glasgow.'

And there was one big consolation. We were going to Sollas, famous among the ambulance pilots for 'Dr Macleod's picnic baskets'. No matter what time of the night or day we landed, there was always a food hamper, prepared by the doctor's wife, waiting for us. And he insisted there was time for a cup of coffee and several of the most succulent meat sandwiches you could taste anywhere before take-off.

It was standard procedure — and the crews appreciated the gesture very much. Certainly it was virtually a life-saver for us that day. We were ravenous when we got to Sollas and I don't think I've ever seen such a wonderful sight as that basket of goodies.

We returned to Renfrew at 7.30pm. It had been a 10-hour day and we were dead-beat. Business tended to be like this. It was either a hunger or a burst. We'd cruise along for a day or two with nothing. Then three or four calls would come in almost together.

A brief log taken from a busy spell I had, will give some idea of the pressure at times.

8 July 1953
0447 — Took off from Renfrew for Barra. Back 2½ hours later.
0830 — Took off for Sollas, North Uist, to bring patient to Renfrew. Back three hours later.
2113 — Answered ambulance call to Campbeltown. Back two hours later.
This meant I was up from three o'clock in the morning until midnight.

9 July 1953
2323 — Called out to Islay. Back at 1.30 the following morning.

11 July 1953
1025 — Answered mercy call to Benbecula. Returned at 2 p.m.

13 July 1953
0340 — Took-off for Benbecula. Back at 0525. Because of radio trouble and bad weather was unable to land to pick up patient.

In that run of six days, I had only one proper night's sleep. I didn't realise how fatigued my body was until we landed back at Renfrew on the morning of the 13th after being forced to call off our mission because of the radio snag and bad weather.

Hoping for a sign that things were clearing-up Benbecula way, we were back and forward to the Met office. Just after 9.00am we were returning from one of these visits when I was conscious of a loud thumping noise. I stopped and said to my radio officer, who had been walking alongside me, 'Do you hear that banging?'

'Aye', he replied, 'I've been wondering what it was.'

You should have seen his face when I told him, 'Well, it's my heart.' It was making a noise like a drum. I went to see the doctor right away. He wrote me out a prescription for some tranquilisers and sent me home to bed.

'The pressure over the past few days has just been too much. You're in danger of straining your heart', he said. Fortunately, the warning had come while I was on the ground and not in the air.

The ambulance case I had been unable to collect was brought in by a Dakota later in the day. I didn't fly again until the 21st. And the few days rest did me the world of good. I've had no similar trouble since.

Extracted from an article which appeared in the Courier & Advertiser *of Dundee in 1968 and reproduced by kind permission of the Editor and of Mrs Sheila Harper (née Barclay).*

A Brush with the Elements

O N THE night of 29th November 1958 fog was playing havoc across the central belt of Scotland. That afternoon Dunfermline's football match against Third Lanark at East End Park had been cancelled — that's how bad it was! As a ghostly grey day turned into eerie darkness still the fog blanketed towns and cities. A late night train from Greenock Princes Pier to Glasgow St Enoch trundled 100 yards past the platform at Kilmacolm before the driver realised that he had missed the station.

Captain Mike O'Brien had no such problems locating North Uist's beach landing strip at Sollas to pick up 81-year-old Angus McAskill. Angus had injured his shoulder in an accident at his home and he was being accompanied by his son on the ambulance flight to hospital in Glasgow. The following morning's press reported 'Mercy Dash in Fog' which, the aircraft crew felt, greatly exaggerated the activities that had occupied their evening.

'How the reporter got to know about it, I don't know', reflected Mike O'Brien, 'but he arrived at Turnhouse Airport with a photographer not long after we had landed. We had a bit of a laugh at the dramatisation but in fact the flight did have its problems.'

'There were no refuelling facilities at Sollas so that when we returned to Glasgow we were rather low on fuel. It was a popular belief that Glasgow and Prestwick were never closed at the same time because of the weather but on this occasion they were both below limits.'

'When we diverted to Turnhouse the weather there was deteriorating and there was not enough fuel left to divert anywhere else so I had to make a landing regardless. In fact we broke out of the cloud exactly at the 'critical height'.'

Mr McAskill was rushed off to Glasgow's Western Infirmary by road ambulance. However the crew were stuck in Edinburgh for the night as was their plane. While they signed off duty and checked into an Edinburgh hotel, a relief crew journeyed through from Renfrew to cover for any ambulance call-outs which would now operate from Turnhouse until the fog in the west started to break up.

Mike O'Brien only undertook occasional ambulance flights during his spell at Renfrew from 1950 until 1961 'helping out to give Captain Barclay days off'. Yet only a few days later, on 9th December, he was again being taunted by the elements in the course of another ambulance flight.

'We departed from Renfrew at 1.15am for Islay. While on the ground a snow storm deposited about three inches of snow on the Heron. There were no de-icing facilities available and a strong easterly wind was blowing. This meant taking off towards the hill and this could be hazardous if the snow didn't blow off during take-off.'

'I called for a broom, climbed up on to the wings and swept the snow off as best I could. All went well.'

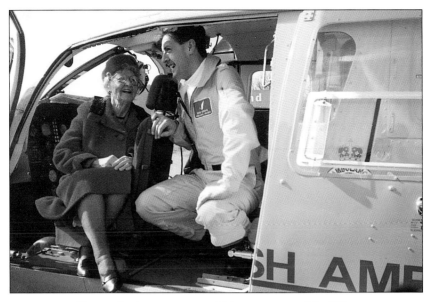

Margaret Boyd compares notes with her counter-part of the 1990s.
(Photo courtesy of Margaret Boyd)

Jonathan Ayres (born on a 'plane) with sister Helen and brother Benjamin in 1992.
(Photo courtesy of Jonathan Ayres)

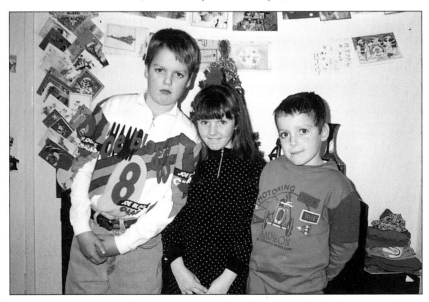

North Uist and Benbecula
Uibhist a' Tuath agus Beinn na Faoghla

✕   Airport / Airstrip

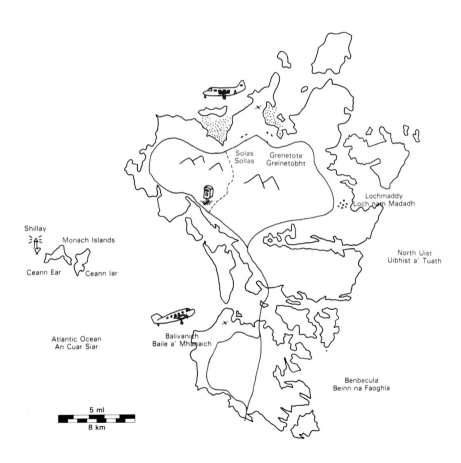

Solas
Sollas

Grenetote
Greinetobht

Lochmaddy
Loch nam Madadh

Shillay

Monach Islands

Ceann Ear   Ceann Iar

North Uist
Uibhist a' Tuath

Balivanich
Baile a' Mhanaich

Atlantic Ocean
An Cuar Siar

Benbecula
Beinn na Faoghla

5 ml
8 km

Orkney

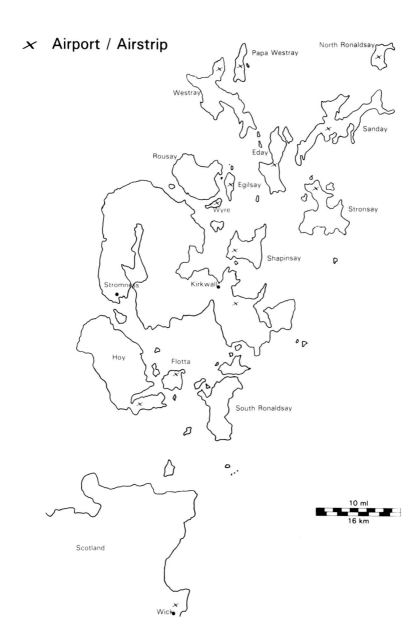

✗ Airport / Airstrip

North Ronaldsay

Papa Westray

Westray

Sanday

Rousay

Eday

Egilsay

Wyre

Stronsay

Shapinsay

Stromness

Kirkwall

Hoy

Flotta

South Ronaldsay

Scotland

Wick

10 ml
16 km

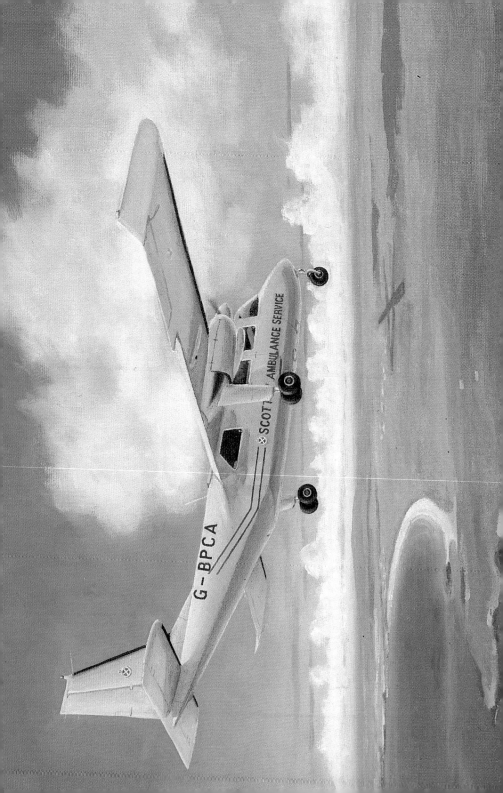

Turn Right at the Post Box

C APTAIN KENNETH McLEAN was based at Renfrew from 1957 until 1961 as a co-pilot on BEA's DC-3 aircraft, called the Pionair class. The DC-3 was the mainstay of the Renfrew fleet which flew the Highlands and Islands routes, but McLean sometimes found himself on the smaller Heron. On one such occasion he found himself on the relief aircraft following the tragic crash on Islay in 1957.

'The Air Ambulance was operated by the de Havilland Heron, flown by a Captain qualified on that type, either accompanied by a Radio Officer, or alternatively by one of the Pionair co-pilots who were not, as far as I now recall, qualified specifically on the Heron. I presume it was certificated for single-pilot operation, so the occupant of the second crew seat was an optional extra, as it were.'

'One such flight that I did was in the company of David Barclay to Sollas, a tiny settlement (village was too grand a title) near the north coast of North Uist. One had to land on the nearby beach, there being just a few airfields — but a lot more beaches — in the Hebrides.'

'The procedure was, first, to fly the approach procedure to Benbecula Airport. This was fairly basic stuff in itself in those days – a "VDF let-down", transmitting by voice on the radio to enable the ground-based operator to obtain and pass back a radio bearing to the pilot. From this the pilot had to figure out what heading to fly to get to where he wanted to be, and as the airfield was getting nearer (so to speak) the requests and replies became virtually a continuous flow of speech, back and forth.'

'One was always glad to have one's calculations and timings confirmed by "engines approaching" or even "engines overhead" from the ground controller who worked in his hut with the door open for just this purpose. How basic can you get? With luck and not a little skill, visual contact with the ground, or sea, would then be made, often in the most marginal conditions.'

'In this case, for Sollas, one then had to follow the road north from Benbecula to North Uist (the A865 on today's maps) and parallel to the west coast for a few miles. At a certain point on that road there was a junction where one turned inland, this junction being recognised by the bright red mail box on a post at the corner; it stood out even in bad weather by virtue of the fact that the surrounding landscape, being treeless, grey and rocky, bore a fair likeness to that of the Moon!'

'From the junction, up over the pass with a very minor road (the Committee Road, David called it) between rocky outcrops, then down the other side, almost straight onto the beach. The patient was loaded on to a flat-bed trailer pulled by an argicultural tractor and brought down to the aircraft that way. I'm sure there were no performance figures for take-off (nor landing); David probably just did it by instinct, having been flying in these conditions in a variety of aircraft for about 30 years by then.'

'He, and other Captains no doubt, had worked out precise and tightly-controlled let-down procedures for some of the places they had to go to in the grimmest weather, using the Decca Navigator system which was fitted to the Herons. This would not be allowed today,

I suspect, but I remember hearing that they would go down to 100 feet over the sea and then make a visual landfall.'

'There certainly is a lot of sea out there, but the adjacent "scenery" is quite unforgiving; that was determination with a capital D, and required a lot of local knowledge and flying skill; one navigated by profile, not plan, on becoming visual. As I was never allowed to fly the aircraft myself in that sort of weather (of course!) I'm sure I can say all that as a tribute to my then mentors without being thought boastful.'

'Stunningly interesting for a pilot, especially looking back from today's rules, regulations and automation; would that I could do it all again!'

Ken Browning flew 168 ambulance flights between 1957 and 1960 and his recollections of Sollas centre around Doctor Alex Macleod of Lochmaddy.

'The trips to Sollas were quite popular, mainly because the doctor, who brought the patient to the beach in his Land Rover, in addition to walking to the edge of the water to indicate the width of beach we had available to land on, and holding his handkerchief in the air to show the wind direction, also brought a basket of goodies; sandwiches, cake and a flask of coffee for us to enjoy. I just hoped the patient didn't mind the extra few minutes wait.'

'There was even a better bonus if you first-footed. I was lucky one New Year when I received a delicious hind-quarter of Hebridean mutton. I have never tasted better.'

'Look what I've got!'

*W*E HAVE an air ambulance call for Barra', said Sister. 'It's a maternity case but no one else is available. Will you take it?'

It was around noon on Sunday, September 1st 1963, and Nurse Isobel Johnstone was supervising lunch in the maternity ward of Glasgow's Southern General Hospital. She was due off at two and looking forward to a lazy afternoon. She had not yet completed even the first part of her midwifery training.

But no nurse ever refuses a call to look after a patient in the air ambulance that plies between Glasgow and the Scottish Highlands and Islands. 'Of course I'll go', she said.

She threw on her cape and hurried across to Home Sister's office. It was probably a mother-to-be, with weeks or even months to go, who needed special treatment in Glasgow. All she would have to do was reassure her during the flight and perhaps treat her for airsickness...

On the windswept island of Barra, Mrs Catherine Gillies, sub-postmistress of the tiny village of Eoligarry, was waiting for the ambulance that would take her to meet the plane.

At forty she was expecting her first baby. Her doctor had foreseen complications and had arranged for her to fly to a Glasgow hospital the following week on an ordinary service plane.

But her labour had started earlier than expected. It was vital that she be moved as quickly as possible. Just before noon, he had called the air ambulance...

— *Air Ambulance* —

In Home Sister's office, Nurse Johnstone picked up the bag of basic medical equipment, together with the special maternity kit, and jumped into the car waiting outside. Within ten minutes, she was at the airport. By twelve-thirty the ambulance plane was on its way.

At Barra she ran across to the waiting ambulance. She still thought it was to be a routine case.

The local district nurse met her. 'The patient's fine', she said, 'She's nicely in labour.'

Nurse Johnstone gasped, 'But I thought...'

'It's all right', said the district nurse reassuringly. 'She'll make it to the mainland.'

The ambulance carried Mrs Gillies across to the plane. As the pilot went through his checks, Nurse Johnstone timed her contractions. They were coming every five minutes. 'I said to the pilot: "She's not going to make it."'

The plane took off into the teeth of the wind. 'It was a wild flight and we were bumping about all over the place.' She glanced down at Mrs Gillies. Her contractions were now coming so quickly. Nurse Johnstone frowned. If there were complications, the nearest help was in Glasgow — still an hour's flight away.

Nurse Johnstone looked at the space around her. The passage was less than three feet wide and the top of the aircraft cabin was almost touching her head. All the things that she had learned in her few months training were about to be put to the test. She would have to deliver the baby here.

'I knew the baby would start to come about a quarter of an hour after take-off, so I broke open the maternity kit. It's sterile and we do this only when birth is imminent. There was no seat or table so I laid out the equipment on the luggage-rack.'

'The mother had been given pain-killing drugs before we left. But she had not been taught how to relax and I had no gas-and-air on board. But I needn't have worried. The baby came after only fifteen minutes. He cried straight away. I felt wonderful.'

'I held him up by the legs and called to the pilot: "Look what I've got!" He was terribly surprised. He'd no idea what had been happening. Then I glanced down at my watch. It was 2.40pm. The pilot said, "We're over Bishopton."'

'The poor wee infant looked very small — he turned out to be five-and-a-half pounds — so I asked the pilot to radio for an oxygen cot to meet us when we landed. I couldn't deliver the afterbirth in case there were complications.'

'There was nowhere to put the baby so I wrapped him in a blanket and then handed him to his mother. She was delighted with herself. "We're calling him Alexander after my husband's father", she said.'

'I made up a bed on the floor and laid Alexander on that. We always keep oxygen on the plane, so I gave him some through a tube in his nose. When we landed, I was sitting in my seat, cuddling him.'

'At the hospital, the doctor said: "You may as well complete the case, Nurse." So I delivered the afterbirth with him looking over my shoulder.'

'I didn't realise that I had done anything unusual until I found a crowd of reporters waiting for me outside the nurses' home.'

When Alexander returned home with his mother, he took with him a very special birth certificate. It has the rare heading 'Air Register Book of Births' and under the first column, 'Registration Marking of Aircraft', is that of the air ambulance, G-ANXB. Date and place of birth are recorded as: 'First day of September 1963. Over Bishopton, Renfrewshire.'

Pilot of the aircraft on which Alexander Gillies was born was Captain Tom Wright. Tom kept in touch with Alexander until he was 21 and remembers the night of his birth well.

'It was another wild day, and flying over the Clyde, Nurse Johnstone came up to the cockpit with a fine baby boy in her arms. I called Air Traffic Control to say that we had gained a passenger during the flight. The Press listened to the control frequency so that, when we landed at Renfrew, they were on to a story. When all the fuss was over we found Nurse Johnstone's midwifery book open at the appropriate page. Miss Johnstone took her final exams a week later and passed with honours.'

Isobel Johnstone had attended air ambulance lectures when she was nearing the end of her second year of training. But she was not permitted to fly until her second year had been completed. She had awaited that time impatiently as she regularly watched third-year friends hurrying off in the airport car, but her first opportunity arrived with greater rapidity than she had anticipated.

'On the very first day of my third year I had the morning off. Around ten, I happened to look out of my room. Sheila, the girl opposite, was getting ready for a flight to Islay. I rushed down to the Home Sister's office. "Can I go too, please?", I asked.'

'She telephoned the airport to see if they could take an observer. "Off you go", she said. Within five minutes I had changed into my uniform and was in the car.'

'When I reached the airport I was scared stiff — the idea of the plane leaving the ground frightened me. This was my first flight and I hadn't thought about it before. We flew over Ardrossan and the Island of Arran. When we got to Islay, we had to circle over the island before landing. The sea looked awfully close. I thought we were going to come down on the water.'

'Our patient was an elderly man with a heart condition. So before we took off, we propped him up and put him on oxygen; and after that he was fine. I soon got over my own fear and I wasn't a bit airsick. But Sheila was sick all the way home. I had to look after both her and the patient.'

'I felt very excited. Now I'd done my observer flight, I wanted to go out again on my own. Every time I was off-duty, I put my name in the book. Within three weeks I'd made seven flights.'

Excitement came thick and fast. 'Ten minutes after starting one flight, I looked out of the window and saw docks and boats. "This is funny", I thought, "We're back in Glasgow." As we landed, I saw fire engines standing by the runway. "What are they for?" I asked the pilot. "Us", he said.'

'When the firemen came on board, he told them there was smoke in the cockpit. It was an hour before we took off again.'

Isobel's greatest satisfaction came from the feeling that she was actually helping to save lives.

'I remember taking off for Islay at eleven o'clock one night. It was for an eight-week-old baby. The doctor had been treating him for a cold but he called around 8 p.m. and didn't like what he saw. When he looked in again at ten, the baby had acute pneumonia.'

'He obviously needed specialised nursing. So the doctor rang up a Glasgow hospital for a bed and called out the air ambulance. We put the baby straight into an oxygen cot on the plane. Within an hour and a half, he was in hospital under care of a paediatrician. The air ambulance had saved that baby's life.'

Sometimes the nurse herself must make the life-or-death decision. Once airborne, she is on her own and for the duration of the trip she has to be nurse, doctor, and consultant combined.

At ten o'clock one Saturday night, Nurse Johnstone was called to Campbeltown. Because of the stretch of water that lies in between, it is 134 miles from Glasgow by road but only sixty by air. This time, the patient was a little girl who had an ulcer and was vomiting blood. The weather was appallingly stormy. The near gale tossed the plane about like a shuttlecock.

'When we landed, the wind caught the aircraft and blew it round. The wing hit the ambulance door. I thought we should still be able to fly back but the pilot said we would have to wait until it could be repaired in the morning.'

"Nurse", he said, "you'll have to take your patient into Campbeltown and wait there."

'I went to see the little girl. She was sick and fretting and looked extremely ill. "She won't wait till morning", I told him. "If she can't fly, I'm taking her to Glasgow by road ambulance."

'We started immediately. It was a wintry night and pitch black. The wind was howling all the way. It took us six hours to get to Glasgow instead of half-an-hour by air. But we made it — and the child's life was saved.'

'That was a time when I didn't wait to ask a doctor's opinion. If the little girl had died, I would have been guilty.'

(Nurse Isobel Johnstone's recollections are taken from an article by Keith Ellis that appeared in Woman magazine in 1964 and they are reproduced with the kind permission of the Editor.)

No Bull

KEITH WARBURTON, now a Training Captain with British Airways on the Boeing 747-400, is yet another captain who began a distinguished flying career on the flight deck of the de Havilland Heron.

'I joined BEA in December 1962 and immediately started the Heron course at Heston with another Flying Officer, Bob Hope. The course consisted of us sitting on either side of the ground instructor with the flying and technical manual between us. Modern day courses are a little different.'

'I commenced flying at the end of January 1963 with Captain Don Hoare. Towards the end of February, with my flying training not fully finished, I went south to visit friends for a few days. On the second day of my absence, frantic telephone messages reached me via my father and Ops at Renfrew. I rang Jimmy Mitchell, who was the Admin Officer for BEA at Renfrew, to find that they wanted me back in Glasgow that night for ambulance stand-by. When I mentioned to Jimmy Mitchell that I hadn't yet completed my training, he said that Captain Barclay had come to the airport and signed me off.'

'Back in Glasgow that night, a phone call to my flat had me off to Islay on my first air ambulance flight. Captain Tom Wright was the captain and I am sure it was a surprise for him to find me as his co-pilot, 22 years old, 200 hours flying and just out of training school.'

'The Heron crews at that time consisted of Training Captains Don Hoare, Ian Montgomery and David Barclay. The Line Captains were Tom Wright, George Ebner, E. Tyrer and G. McLean; assisted by Flying Officers Gordon, Stewart, Dowling and myself.'

'As the Heron was very small there was no catering facility on board. We therefore took a picnic box which was prepared for us, both for ambulances and scheduled services, by the aircraft caterers at Renfrew Airport. If one was flying with Captain Barclay he would arrive at briefing, have a quick look at the weather, then leave the co-pilot to do all the flight planning while he went off to see the ladies in the kitchen about the picnic box.'

'Also because of the space limitations, the Heron had no toilet on board. Captain Barclay had a rather weak bladder and had to use a sick bag. He was always very apologetic about having to use it when accompanied by any co-pilot for the first time.'

'One night in a local pub near Renfrew, most of the Heron co-pilots were having a drink when one mentioned the use of the sick bag and how Captain Barclay always waited until he got over a particular island before opening the window and throwing it out. Next day I was flying with him and the usual routine happened. He waited until we were over the island and then out went the bag. I just couldn't resist asking why he always waited until reaching this point. He reply was, "Because I cannae stand the Duke of Argyll." *

'Upon another occasion we were departing from Barra, where we had had our picnic, to Tiree. As we taxied out there was a bullock on the beach. I suggested to him that we should go back and get Donald, the fireman, to chase him off. But Captain Barclay decided that we could do it with the aircraft. Having moved the animal to one end, we were ready for take-off.'

'Captain Barclay knew that I had my camera with me and told me to have it ready. We were about two feet off the beach as we rushed passed the bullock. Sometime later I brought the photographs in to show him. He was highly delighted with the shot of the bullock on the beach and immediately took it to show Captain Starling (the boss). I thought my career was over.'

'On another occasion we went to Shetland, a place which by then he rarely visited. He was quite upset because a lot of his old friends had passed away since his last visit. Because it was a fairly urgent ambulance case, we flew straight back to Aberdeen. I asked what height to flight plan at and he said we would go visually. I reminded him that the cloud base was 800 feet so he said we would go at 500 feet!'

'On the way down to Aberdeen, Captain Barclay tucked into the picnic while I flew the aircraft. When he had finished, it was my turn to eat. As he got some food out for me he discovered that we had run out of napkins — so he stuffed the met chart on to the front of my shirt.'

'One day during a turnaround at Renfrew, a reporter had come to interview him. He wasn't very keen until he learned that he would get a fee for it. I was sworn to secrecy not to tell his wife about the fee. Captain Barclay was a great chap to fly with. He was most generous and helpful and it was a privilege for me to have flown in his company.'

'When we flew to Benbecula, Dr Macleod always met us with a picnic unless it was an emergency. One day we arrived there and it was so windy that we could not turn off the runway. So we remained there and the ambulance came out to us. But the wind was so strong we were unable to open the aircraft door outwards so as to manoeuvre the stretcher aboard.'

'The fire engine had to be called so that it could park across the aircraft nose and break the airflow over the aircraft and therefore the pressure on the door so that we could load the stretcher.'

'I was on ambulance standby one Sunday morning with Tom Wright when we received an urgent call to go to Barra where fortunately the tide was suitable for a landing. I drove to the airport as fast as I could and nearly hit Tom Wright as we simultaneously turned into the car park.'

'We rushed to the aircraft and found the nurse from the Southern General waiting for us. The flight was quite rough and she was sick en route. On arrival at Barra, a Sunday morning, everybody was there to meet us in Sunday suits. Among them was Donald, the fireman, on the tender in his best suit.'

'The ambulance had been called for the post-mistress who was expecting a baby. Since the first signs had begun and the lady was 40, it was felt that hospital was the best place. Unfortunately the baby didn't wait and was born during the flight. At one stage I thought I was going to have to go back to help as the nurse was still feeling sick. It was headline news in the next day's papers.'

* Geoff Northmore, who flew as First Officer with David Barclay during 1959/60, remembers this habit, 'We First Officers reckoned we could find the route to fly by following the trail of discarded sickness bags.'

Sad visit to Tiree

NURSE LESLEY CRAWFORD undertook her first ambulance flight in 1964 from her base at Glasgow's Southern General Hospital.

'Before flying on the air ambulance we were given two training lectures. They were really quite basic courses of instruction. The first gave us basic information about our nursing duties in the aircraft and special procedures that we might have to follow in specific medical cases. The second course covered procedures in an emergency when the patient no longer remained the responsibility of the nurse but became that of the captain of the aircraft.'

'At all other times the nurse was responsible for the welfare of the patient totally because there was no doctor in attendance. Only a nurse resident at the hospital could register to be on standby and her bag was always kept at the ready. The equipment that it contained was really quite basic. Another air ambulance nurse would accompany you on your first flight but after that you were on your own. Many of the girls had never flown before joining the air ambulance. Air sickness could be a problem for the nurses and of course the patient might also have air sickness added to his other ailments.'

Lesley flew on the de Havilland Herons of BEA and recalls how attentive the pilots always were. 'The captain always checked the inside of the cabin thoroughly before we set off, and the first officer would often come back and join me during the outward flight when we were going to collect a patient.' Lesley obviously relished the consideration that the flight crew gave her but ensuring that their nurse was given full courtesy and attention can only have a been a pleasure to them.

'The air ambulance planes were small and this was real flying. The air ambulance pilots who flew them were masters of their craft and could handle them with extreme dexterity.'

The mission that Lesley remembers most vividly has remained in her memory because it was not a happy one. The air ambulance crew had been called to Tiree to collect an extremely sick baby.

'When the road ambulance arrived at Reef Aerodrome a very young mother alighted carrying her small white bundle and she handed the baby to me. It was very, very still and when I looked at it I could see no signs of life. The doctor had been following by car and when he arrived I immediately had him examine the baby which he certified as dead. The poor infant must have died just minutes before reaching the aerodrome. The news had to be broken to the mother who was inconsolable and we flew back to Renfrew heavy-hearted and without a patient.'

Landing at Barra, where the aircraft would sweep over the house of writer Compton MacKenzie to touch down on the sands, is always a memorable experience. 'The regular passenger flights always landed at low tide but on ambulance flights we sometimes had to touch down in a few inches of water. Welly boots were an integral part of my equipment upon those occasions.'

Lesley Crawford never had to deliver a baby in flight, a circumstance which she recalls with relief, 'But I had some near misses.'

Many of her colleagues volunteering for ambulance flights were from the islands. 'Because of the close-knit communities of the islands, many nurses had friends or relatives who had had to use the air ambulance at some time and they were most often taken to the Southern General. It therefore followed that when island girls decided to take up a career in nursing, the Southern General was the hospital to which they first applied. A strong bond between the hospital and the Hebrides therefore developed over the years.'

'Doctors would select the hospital to which they wanted their patient to go. It therefore followed that if an island G.P. had trained at the Western Infirmary or the Royal Infirmary, he would have colleagues there and an affinity with that hospital. Most cases came to the Southern General but the choice was always that of the local island doctor.'

Lesley Crawford's air ambulance flying terminated when promotion took her to Canniesburn Hospital, Glasgow. Now retired, she is still reminded of the occasion when she was awarded her air ambulance wings when she occasionally sees an air ambulance helicopter come in to land near her home at Fort Matilda, or an Islander fly up the Clyde estuary towards the city. 'If it's flying low, I never have to wonder the reason why.'

The Night of the Blue Lights

*I*T WAS an inky black November night, incessant rain being driven by an unrelenting wind, when I met Nurse Co-ordinator Islay Skea before she began her shift through the night at Glasgow's Southern General Hospital.

She had just received word that a Search and Rescue (SAR) Sea King helicopter was expected at the hospital helipad and she was not looking forward to providing a reception on the ground while the helicopter's rotors whipped the puddles and falling rain into a frenzy. But that time was not yet imminent. Messages were being relayed to her office as we chatted, with the news that the helicopter was detained on the ground at Loch Long and was not yet able to lift off with its patient, an injured soldier, because of the inclement weather.

During recent years Islay Skea has been involved with the air ambulance service in a variety of ways. These include co-ordinating nurses for air ambulance duties, putting aspiring air ambulance volunteers through their specialist training for taking to the air, and addressing various groups and organisations anxious to know more about the service.

But the prevailing stormy weather on this November night took her back to one of her own very first flights, on board a BEA Heron bound for Campbeltown in January 1965.

'We took off from Renfrew just before 5.00pm and flew straight into a gale. Lightning was streaking across the sky, then suddenly a blue flash ran right through the cockpit. We had been hit!'

'The force of the lightning strike abruptly knocked the aircraft higher into the sky and my ears felt numb with the sudden change in pressure.'

'I felt unable to hear, but was greatly relieved when Captain Wakefield called to me from the flight deck to enquire if I was all right.'

'It was so reassuring because I was wondering if he was all right as I was sure that the lightning had passcd right through the aircraft.'

'We continued our journey and as we came into land I noticed that blue lights were flashing on the ground. It was normal for a fire tender to stand by when we came in to land, but this time there was also an ambulance and there were too many lights for Campbeltown.'

'Until now I had been unaware that we had turned back to Renfrew, the Heron's compass having been rendered useless by the bolt of lightning, and we were the focus of a full emergency alert.'

'The Press were later to report me as a heroine who had declined the offer of a replacement nurse for a second attempt. I don't recall ever being given the option, but I do recall the privilege of a cup of tea in the airport cafeteria. Such refreshment was usually restricted to a chipped enamel mug in the informal surroundings of the ops room.'

'When we took off again it was in the larger Handley Page Herald and I couldn't help noticing that I had a different pilot and co-pilot. When we reached Campbeltown the patient was quite irate at being kept waiting for so long.'

'I got him settled on the aircraft but he insisted in being sat at the window with the blind up so that he could watch the lightning. After my earlier experience I was in favour of having the blind securely down. When I was a child lightning used to fascinate me, but since that night I now always feel nervous about lightning.'

'The patient, suffering from an abdominal complaint, was delivered to the Western Infirmary. It was about midnight when I returned to the Southern General. Earlier I had injured my leg in the operating theatre so I went to have it seen to and emerged wearing an impressive bandage.'

'If a nurse had undergone a bad experience on a flight, it was customary to get her back in the air as quickly as possible in case she was deterred from further flying. So next day I found myself going on another flight, this time to Islay. With my leg bandaged, I looked as much an invalid as my patient.'

'That flight was in a Vickers Viscount, a 70-passenger plane and I had it all to myself. BEA's Robert McKean met me upon our return to Renfrew and he gave me a small card that was issued to certify each ambulance flight undertaken by a nurse. I remember him commenting that I'd now flown on the whole fleet.'

'The Press interest continued for 48 hours and the journalists were taken in hand by the Matron. When I returned late at night from the Campbeltown flight I remember her coming out in dressing gown and slippers. I had only ever seen her in the formality of her well-pressed uniform and had never imagined her in slippers.'

'I recall insisting that I should be credited with two flights for Campbeltown. I was just 22 and was anxious to gain my Wings. But I was firmly told that I had only brought in one patient, so it was one flight!'

Captain Mac and the Boy from Mull

C APTAIN DUNCAN McINTOSH, known affectionately as 'Captain Mac' to his colleagues, founded Loganair in 1962 and ran the airline for 21 years. While his duties kept him behind a desk more and more as the airline grew, he would climb into the cockpit whenever the opportunity or the need arose. This was particularly true of ambulance flights as he recalled one busy week.

'In seven days not so long ago, I flew six mercy missions, three from Coll, one from Mull and two from Oronsay.'

'The Mull call came in late one Saturday evening. It was very bad weather when I flew out from Glasgow and I had difficulty finding the island. I had no way of knowing how serious the case was. It was touch and go, but I managed to land as darkness was closing in.'

'The patient was an 11-month-old boy who was dangerously ill. He had swallowed the head of a plastic soldier which had bristles on it. It was blocking the windpipe and he was being given oxygen.'

'His condition was so serious that the doctor came back to Glasgow with us. The youngster needed oxygen all the way to keep him alive.'

'On the way his condition deteriorated. I radioed Abbotsinch for emergency clearance to land. Air traffic control were extremely helpful. They gave me permission to land on the nearer short runway to save going round the main runway. There was only one snag. The short runway was unlit. So they illuminated it with car headlights.'

'An ambulance with police car escort was waiting and I managed to stop the Islander in a very short distance right beside them. Our patient was rushed with police escort to the Southern General Hospital.'

'As they were taking him from the ambulance, he died. He had suffered what is known as cardiac arrest.'

'Because he was so close to the operating theatre, however, they managed to whip him in and get the heart started again.'

'The drama wasn't over. He was transferred to the Oakbank Children's Hospital where operations are carried out. There it was discovered the obstruction had passed down to the heart valve and was blocking one side of the heart.'

'The operation was successful. Next day he was eating his breakfast, right as rain. Later the doctor told me that if we had been two minutes later, there would have been no hope of saving the child's life.'

'I got a very nice letter from the islanders for helping to save the life of this little boy and an earlier patient, a girl suffering from pleurisy.'

Extracted from an interview which appeared in the Courier and Advertiser of Dundee in 1970 and reproduced by kind permission of the Editor.

Islander on Orkney

*A*RTHUR KERR joined the RAF in 1942, gaining his wings in Canada and becoming well immersed in the propeller aircraft of the time. His service culminated with flying off Malta, during which time the first marine salvage claim registered by an air crew was lodged. The claim was submitted with a degree of humour and produced a salvage fee of £50. After a spell in commerce, Arthur turned to commercial flying, on the flight deck of the Airspeed Ambassadors of Autair International Airways and BAC 1-11 jets of Court Line.

'This required a lot of night flying and when I tired of spending summer days catching up on my sleep, I joined Loganair, based in Orkney. This was in July 1970 and I succeeded Barney Barron. Barney was another ex-Fleet Air Arm pilot. It seemed at that time that Loganair consisted mainly of ex-RAF or ex-Fleet Air Arm pilots and we all seemed to have 1939-45 or Korean War medal ribbons. There are few of those about now.'

'Ken Foster was my instructor, converting me on to the Islander. My first flight upon arrival in Orkney was to fly an ambulance case to Aberdeen. The nurse was Elsie Setter, and it was one of what I regarded as hair-raising flights compared to my normal route flying on a BAC 1-11 at 37,000 feet. I probably shouldn't describe it this way, but for an elderly pilot it was quite a new experience.'

'Route training in Orkney required six landings on each of the scheduled landing strips. I was taken on a quick hurl round one fine day doing the requisite number of landings on each island. I was then a line pilot. There were no navigational aids except for a VOR at Kirkwall. There was a type of NDB which was really the lighthouse transmitting and one could get a bearing off Sanday lighthouse every so many minutes. This was fine for the first couple of days in clear visibility but in a short time the scheduled run was being made in rather poor weather. Not knowing all the local landmarks I soon got lost. So I threw the chart to the passengers with, ''You've been here more often than me, so show me where we are and we'll carry on.''

'But I soon built up a store of information, tide demarcation marks, red barn doors, lines of telegraph poles, a broken down tractor in a field, or a particular coastal rock formation. Navigation quickly became a case of reading the landmarks. Getting bearings and fixes by radio signals was inappropriate to the short distances. Fair Isle, only served on a charter basis at that time, was a tricky landing and was often at the whim of the direction of the wind.'

'Late one winter's day I had to fly a woman patient, in the company of her husband, from Orkney to Aberdeen. The husband seemed to be more excited about flying than he was about his wife's condition. On the return journey the weather was deteriorating as we left the Banffshire coast and we were flying in VFR conditions which gradually became untenable. The cloud base became so low that we were below the cliff level, making it difficult to find the way. Not knowing what might lie ahead I began climbing to about 8,000 feet and the VOR readings became a bit unreliable.'

'As I was unsure of the readings that I was getting, I made a call to Rosehearty Radar for a position report. They identified me as being at about 130 miles over the Bay of

Kirkwall. There was no alternative but to start a descent. I picked up the Kirkwall VOR to get confirmation of my position and I did a slow circular descent at that position, cautious in the knowledge of the high ground at Hoy and at Wideford. But Rosehearty was absolutely spot on. We broke cloud at about five or six hundred feet right over the Bay of Kirkwall. From there it was just a case of following the coastline to Kirkwall Airport.'

'The flight was concluded with me glad to be back safely on firm ground. However my passenger showed no concern at all and seemed to think that he was immortal, saying how thoroughly he had enjoyed the flight. He obviously didn't realise how much my faith had been in the radar rather than in my own skills.'

'Inaugural mail runs to the Northern Isles took place on 23rd November 1970 and I took the first mail flight to Eday. Eday was a difficult one if you didn't know your way around. We landed on Loch London which was a dried up sand bed. There were patches of quicksand and one night I took a wrong turning off the landing strip and ended up with the nose wheel of the Islander buried up to its axle in soft sand. There was a nurse on board and she took control so that in a very few minutes a tractor appeared and got us out of the sand. She took photographs of the incident which proved embarrassing as she sent them to the flight office afterwards.

'Another embarrassing incident, in my early days with Loganair, occurred on Stronsay. The airfield sloped to the west and had been created by making a gap in a dyke. I was not very familiar with the layout of the field and just as I landed, the clouds opened and mud quickly spattered on to the windscreen so that I couldn't see anything except a pair of markers. I thought that they marked the end of the field but they seemed to have come up far too quickly. I looked out of the small inspection window at the side of the aircraft to see that it was the long arm of the stone dyke. I tried to make a quick turn but caught the Islander's port oleo on the dyke. The aircraft came to an abrupt halt and settled on the ground with the deadly quiet that follows such situations. In view of the absence of windscreen wipers on the Islander and my newness to the strip, I was exonerated from any blame in this incident. I'm sure that I was not the only pilot to bend aeroplanes on the basic Orkney strips.'

'All of the landing strips were fields, sometimes two knocked into one by removing stone dyking. They were covered in mud and sharn. This threw up on to the windscreen on take-off so that you were almost blind-flying by the time you were airborne. We had no windscreen wipers so we would look for a rain cloud in the hope that the rain would wash off the sharn. The sharn also got into the air intakes for the aircraft heating systems where it began to cook and fill the aircraft with a pretty foul stench at times. A rain coat and wellingtons were standard uniform in winter when the airfields were extremely muddy.'

'Rabbits dug their burrows in the landing strips too, especially on Sanday where I landed one night to take a patient to Kirkwall. Tractors stood with their headlights pointing down-wind and we landed into the lights. These always took place in at least semi-moonlight conditions. When I turned out of the glare of the tractor lights, the aircraft lights picked up hundreds and hundreds of eyes staring at me, Sanday's rabbit population.'

'One elderly woman being taken to hospital in Kirkwall was taken to the airfield at Westray with great difficulty. She was having none of these new-fangled motor vehicles. She had no qualms about boarding the plane, but upon arrival at Kirkwall Airport new problems arose when she refused to board the ambulance that was to take her to Balfour Hospital.'

'Andy Alsop, Loganair's Chief Pilot in Orkney for many years, looked on the operation as his own. He was very media-minded and never missed a trick to get Loganair into the press. He was probably Loganair's best ambassador in the Seventies. For my part, I moved back to the BAC 1-11 when I could no longer stand the noise of the Islander's engines!'

Combined Effort on Unst

A LAN WHITFIELD served with Loganair for 13 years starting in 1969. The first ten of these were spent in the Shetland Islands where he built up a network of island airfields.

The most northerly Shetland airfield is Unst and it was here, at a latitude of 60°45N, in 1972, that he landed in almost impossible conditions thanks to the provision of communications equipment of abnormal sophistication — the result of a very informal arrangement.

'In March I had to carry out a particularly difficult ambulance flight, one which would have been impossible without the co-operation of the RAF at Saxa Vord, about six miles away at the extreme north of Unst. I received a call at about 2330 hours to say that a man on Unst had suffered a heart attack and the doctor wished to evacuate him to hospital as soon as possible. The weather was poor but not impossible, so I agreed to have a go with the proviso that I would not try to land at Tingwall, Lerwick's local airfield, because, with the state of the weather, I was doubtful of attempting to fly into the valley that night. It would save time if the road ambulance came straight to Sumburgh, 28 miles to the south, to await my return.'

'It was a very dark night, with the cloud base at about 600 feet, as I set course northwards. I flew just off the coast, maintaining my distance by watching the phosphorescence of the waves breaking on the rocks. It was clear enough to see the light beacon on Mousa and, as I passed it, I would see the lights of Lerwick ahead. I passed over the harbour at Lerwick leaving Bressay to my right and, as I cleared the north entrance of Bressay Sound, I could see the light flashing on the pier at Symbister on Whalsay. I therefore felt confident of reaching Unst without too much trouble.'

'After Whalsay there would be no more lights until I reached Unst and, if it was very dark, I would then veer to the east to track over the lighthouse on Out Skerry. From there I would set course for Unst, secure in the knowledge that I would pass to the east of Fetlar and so getting a clear run in to Unst where a small light beacon some two miles east of the airstrip would give me some guidance.'

'Unst had no air radio beacon at that time but limited guidance could be obtained from a maritime radio beacon on Muckle Flugga, the most northerly inhabited point in the British Isles, lying about six miles north of the airstrip. I could only obtain a bearing from this beacon for two minutes in every six as it was one of a cycle of beacons which transmit in turn from various locations so that a ship can take cross bearings for a position fix. This is fine for a sea vessel with lots of time to plot the position but of no real value for finding the airstrip in an aeroplane.'

'However I had a highly unofficial arrangement with the lighthouse keeper that, in a dire emergency, he would switch the beacon onto continuous transmit by holding the cycling mechanism closed thereby giving me a steady bearing to home onto. I was also able to use the distance element of a military navigation system, TACAN, which was installed at Saxa Vord to give me a continuous readout of my distance from the transmitter.'

'The end of the runway on Unst was 6.2 miles from this beacon and, by using a combination of these two systems, I knew that I could reach the approximate end of the runway — but not with sufficient accuracy to make an instrument approach, hence the need to fly maintaining visual contact.'

'Soon after passing over the Out Skerries I realised that the cloud was getting too low to continue underneath it so I was forced to climb to a safe height. At about 1,000 feet I came out of the cloud into clear sky to see a most fantastic sight. There was an aurora that night which was particularly bright and the top of the cloud layer was bathed in a luminous green light. Whilst this was most spectacular, I was not very happy about the brightness as I knew that, when I finally descended into the murk below the cloud, my vision would take time to adapt to the darkness.

'At that time we could talk to the RAF controller at Saxa Vord so I asked him to implement the arrangement with the lighthouse keeper and soon my radio direction finder was pointing steadily towards Muckle Flugga. This enabled me to home in overhead and set course in an easterly direction until my distance measuring equipment, tuned to Saxa Vord, showed that I was approaching the six-mile point.'

'I then started to fly a curving path to the right, holding the distance at 6.2 miles and descending to the lowest safe height at which I could fly on instruments without danger of flying into the hill to the west of the airstrip. At this height I was still in cloud and eventually, when I knew I must be over the strip, I had to overshoot and climb back above the cloud.'

'As I passed over the strip I noticed a glow in the cloud which I assumed was the RAF fire engine shining its searchlight straight upwards. This was confirmed to me by the Saxa Vord controller calling me up to say that the fire crew had heard me pass overhead. He also informed me that the patient's condition had deteriorated rapidly and that the doctor was very anxious to know what I thought of my chances of getting in.'

'I explained my difficulties to the controller with regard to the cloud base and the absence of any means of establishing the location of the end of the strip. At this, another voice came on the radio which I recognised as belonging to the senior controller whom I knew quite well. He asked me if I was sure that I could identify the airstrip from above the cloud. I agreed to try so I asked that once again the fire engine should shine its searchlight straight up and fire off flares as I passed over.'

'I repositioned myself to the east and approached again without descending into the cloud. I soon spotted the glow of the light and called for a flare. A few moments later it soared up out of the cloud giving me a positive position.'

'Whilst I was doing this the controller had been watching me on the large air defence radar which normally searched to the north and east for Soviet aircraft. He now had the position of the strip marked on the radar screen and asked if I would like to try a sort of ground-controlled approach with his very unofficial assistance. I agreed to this, asking him to overshoot me one mile before I reached the coast if I didn't have visual contact. In the meantime the fire crew down at the strip passed on a weather observation giving me the visibility at 1,500 yards and the cloud base at about 250 feet. It was going to be very tight!'

'I again positioned to the east and, obtaining steering courses from the radar controller, started to descend, deciding that I would go down to 200 feet if necessary. Lower than that would be hazardous unless I was in the clear beneath the cloud. At 300 feet the sea was just becoming visible so I continued down to 250 feet which put me just below the cloud. Visibility ahead was very poor due to a steady drizzle but, with the radar controller giving me a continuous distance to go, I continued.'

'Out of the gloom, the small light beacon on Balta, the island to the east of Baltasound, loomed up and, as I passed it, I saw the glow of the searchlight on the fire engine. Then the gooseneck flares along the edges of the strip appeared. I put down full flap and landed, calling the controller as I did so in order that the radar and the lighthouse beacon could revert to their official functions.'

'We loaded the patient and a doctor and soon took off again for Sumburgh. The patient survived and next day was transferred to a hospital on the mainland. So ended what must be a unique event in three-way co-operation and probably the only instance in which a huge long range air defence radar has been turned round to provide a GCA approach!'

'Ambulance flying, or indeed any other sort of emergency or Search & Rescue flying, has to be a very carefully balanced operation. Great care must be taken not to let the drama of the situation cloud one's judgement. Indeed a healthy sense of fear is perhaps the single most useful attribute in these situations. There is no place for the ''steely eyed and lantern jawed'' character so beloved of movie producers. Such a one would inevitably end up with a broken aeroplane, if not worse, and this is of no use to the patient who is lying waiting for the aircraft's arrival.'

'I was also aware of the nurse riding in the back and trusting in me to get her safely back to the hospital with her patient, and of my own family at home who wanted me back safely. Every move had to be thought out ahead of time, a course of action decided which would cover any eventuality, and a firm decision made, when the conditions were too bad, to turn around and try again later. This philosophy enabled me to carry out over five hundred such flights safely. There was only one occasion when I was unable to complete a mission although there were some cases where I had to make two or three attempts before succeeding.'

Corrigan's Kippers

*J*OHN CORRIGAN served with Scottish Airways, BEA, and British Airways from 1945 until 1980. With BEA and British Airways he was Group Supervisor Technical Services, and Engineering Quality Control Supervisor for their Scottish-based aircraft. These included Hawker Siddeley 748s of British Airways, Handley Page Dart Heralds of BEA — and the de Havilland Herons. John's work included routine maintenance, modifications, development, Certificate of Airworthiness renewals, and test flights. The planning of maintenance and physical involvement were combined with liaison with other airline departments and with the aircraft manufacturers.

'The Air Ambulance Herons were my particular babies. Overhaul of our aircraft would normally be organised and certificated by staff in our Inspection Department, but this facility was closed in the middle of 1956. Because of my licence coverage for airframe overhaul in addition to engines and also because of previous Inspection Branch experience, these tasks now fell to me.'

'The job demanded most of my time, including off-duty hours at all times of the day and night. My wife supported me completely, enduring many phone calls from various parties — engineering, operations, etc., asking for advice or authority from me on a technical or other problem which could not wait. One could not always return to bed easily and often it meant going into work to solve the problem. Engineering "wags" eventually referred to the Herons as "Corrigans Kippers". I took it as a compliment!'

'I monitored their progress during construction in the de Havilland factory at Chester 1954-55, accepted them on completion on behalf of BEA and looked after them in every conceivable engineering respect for 18 years 9 months before eventually delivering them to Peters Aviation, Norwich, in 1973, after we relinquished the Air Ambulance Contract. It was like handing over a large part of my life.'

'The engineers, aircrew, nurses, outstation staff and de Havilland staff I worked with throughout that long period, and the end product of our combined efforts, made those 18 years the most satisfying of my entire working life. We had many problems, engineering, defect investigation, planning, operational and administrative, providing ambulance cover 365 days a year. Occasionally two call-outs overlapping as well as regular Heron passenger services to the Outer Isles with only two aircraft to do the job (having lost a third aircraft in the crash of 1957) placed extraordinary demands upon us. We always managed, because of the extra effort everyone always provided at the mention of Air Ambulance. Strikes never affected us and we had unique ways of ensuring that we never had both aircraft grounded for maintenance at the same time, and if by some unavoidable circumstance they were, we ensured one at least could be ready for the crew within the time it took the crew and nurse to reach the airport from their homes and the Southern General Hospital.'

'The distinctive drone of the Heron's four engines at night, climbing away from Renfrew or Abbotsinch, over Clydebank and the Kilpatrick Hills, became as familiar to my wife and family as they were to me — one of "my" Herons was off to the Isles — for someone in need.'

'Another type of co-operation and motivation that we all had is illustrated by an incident at Barra. On landing approach to the beach a Heron clipped a sand dune, damaging No. 2 prop tip, port fuselage, side skin and port inner flap. With three engineers and some "guessed at" spares, we proceeded to Barra in the other Heron with seats out to accommodate the new flap and spares. Unloading and seat transference at Barra was very rapid. Then our relief aircraft resumed the service leaving us with the damaged aircraft.'

'The weather was rapidly worsening with the tide about to turn, so — with visions of a Rapide that years previously was trapped in similar circumstances, and no time to lose — we removed the damaged No. 2 prop and blanked it off, changed the damaged flap, with the wind, rain and sea spray half blinding us. "Labouring" assistance and hot drinks were provided by crew and local staff as we patched the damaged fuselage skin with a large panel, blind rivetted for speed. It was a factory prefabricated panel, complete with bonded stringers, so for quickness yet strength retention, we fitted it "inside out", stringers exposed.'

'The crew made a perfect three-engine take-off, from a standing start on a rapidly diminishing beach and we were on our way home, chilled but thrilled! During the trip I sat next to the fuselage repair "to keep an eye on it" and the slipstream whistling through the stringers made an unholy screaming noise like a miniature Stuka dive bomber — but it held together. Permanent repairs back home saw the aircraft back in service within twenty-four hours.'

'Aircraft visiting Barra's beach had to be hosed down with fresh water every day to remove salt, but the corrosive action was still severe, so the keel panels on both aircraft, plus many alloy components, were renewed several times over the years. Series 1B Herons were chosen for their fixed undercarriage, which was stronger than the Series 2A's retractable undercarriage, and more suitable for rough strips and better cross-wind component. Experimenting at one time for a suitable landing area on Coll had drastic results — no injuries, but the aircraft was severely damaged. It had to be dismantled on site, then engines, mainplanes, fuselage, etc., towed on trailers to the nearest beach on a tank landing-craft. It then continued by sea and road to the de Havilland factory where it had major repairs, including a complete immersion bath in fresh water. It was out of service for several months, during which time we hired another Heron and it was the only time we did not have the capacity to do our own repairs.'

'G-AOFY was our third Heron, bought some time after 'XA and 'XB. It was lost at Islay in 1957 with Paddy Calderwood, captain, Hugh McGinlay, first officer, and Sister Jean Kennedy all giving their lives in a valiant attempt to uplift a very sick patient in atrocious weather. I flew with Paddy and Hugh many times and can still "see" them.'

'The Herons were modified in several ways to suit their ambulance duties. To accommodate certain heart patients and other medical conditions where the stretcher had to be kept as flat as possible at all times, including during loading and unloading, necessitated fitting a "false" secondary level floor to the rear cargo hold because the original one was on a slope. Also, as there was no auto pilot fitted and the pilots had to fly "hands on" as steady as possible in all kinds of weather, we had to maintain the controls rigging as accurate as possible at all times. A special patient/stretcher support unit was made with various medical equipment compartments, in collaboration with the Southern General Hospital, to keep the patient secure and at an agreeable height beside the nurse. A glass fibre nose wheel mudguard was designed and fitted to reduce the nose wheel "bow wave" which previously shot straight on to No. 2 and 3 engines when landing and taking off at Barra beach with its many puddles. Many modifications and continuous development went on over the years.'

'We were always supported by our General Services section producing ground equipment, for handling aircraft ambulance equipment as well as passenger equipment, cargo equipment, outstation fire fighting equipment, etc. produced by joiners, painters, electricians, and others. The General Services Manager, Bill Young, who had started his career as an aircraft electrician, tragically died at an early age. I had the honour to agree to Mrs Young's request to scatter Bill's ashes over the Firth of Clyde from the air. We arranged it should be done on a Glasgow homeward leg, the outward leg being a patient being delivered home.'

'There was no precedent, so I had to select a suitable existing aperture on the Heron fuselage, slightly modify it, design and make a suitable funnel to combat the slipstream and hopefully create a slight venturi effect. When a suitable occasion arose, the BEA nurse accompanied me with Bill's ashes and mid-way over the Firth of Clyde at about 3,500 feet the skipper throttled back to minimum control speed while we slowly consigned Bill's ashes to the elements. It was a beautiful sunny afternoon. Prestwick and the Ayrshire coast lay ahead, Arran and Holy Isle behind, the Trossachs to the left, and Ailsa Craig to the right. I still stop occasionally on the Dunure road and view the scene. I said a few words I had prepared, wished his soul peace, and thanked the Lord for his comradeship while with us. It was a humbling experience, and yet another unforgettable link forged with the Herons.'

'We finally sold the Herons to Peters Aviation of Norwich in 1973. Well maintained, with low hours for their age, they were a bargain. In September 1973 'XA did a two-month charter in West Africa with Sierra Leone Airways before delivery to Peters Aviation — quite a change of climate after 18 years around the Scottish islands.'

'BEA's two long-serving Herons concluded their 18 years with the airline having each flown approximately 2 million miles. Coincidentally their de Havilland serial numbers closely matched their total hours flown, while their landing frequency shows that the average flight time was about 45 minutes:

G-ANXB	Serial No	14,048	accepted 12 February 1955
	Flying hours	14,505	at 15 October 1973
	Landings	18,368	at 15 October 1973
G-ANXA	Serial No	14,044	accepted 23 February 1955
	Flying hours	14,163	at 20 November 1973
	Landings	18,973	at 20 November 1973'

Herons to Mach 2

C APTAIN VIVIAN GUNTON joined BEA in 1962 straight from training at Hamble, the first captain to join the state corporation from this source. He flew his first flight in command of the Heron on 31st March 1970 and was to log up nearly 1,000 hours on the type in less than three years.

'The first time I was called up at night for an ambulance was a new experience for me. The telephone rang. I picked up the receiver, turned on the light, and looked at the clock. It indicated 3.00am. I put the phone down, turned the light off and put my head back on the pillow. I almost went back to sleep but my wife elbowed me and said, "Who was that?" I said, "It's probably the Company." She said, "What time are you going out then?" At which point I sat bolt upright in bed, grabbed for the telephone, dialled the airport number which was engaged. I think the Duty Officer was still sitting there with his jaw agape wondering what he was supposed to do now, having got that response from the ambulance captain. When I did get through, he was terribly polite about it. "Some problem with the phones, Captain."'

'This reminds me of an incident involving David Jones who lived in Kilbarchan and another captain who lived in Bridge of Weir. It was the middle of the night with freezing conditions. David was driving from Kilbarchan and reached the top of the hill that descends on to the Bridge of Weir to Paisley road. He put his foot on the brakes and nothing happened. He carried on down the hill conscious of a car approaching from Bridge of Weir. Fortunately that car accelerated and he was able to slide across the junction, miss the back of it, hit the gutter and then follow the other car to the airport.'

'The other captain reported that he was driving along the road and he could see lights coming down the hill at a very constant speed. He accelerated slightly and a car slid across behind him, hit the gutter, and then followed him to the airport. The two of them wondered quite how the Duty Officer would have coped with the air ambulance call-out if they had pranged into each other.'

'Severe conditions were a hazard in the air too. I once saw rain-ice falling on the aeroplane which, at the sort of levels and temperatures at which we were operating the Heron in Scotland, was a bit disconcerting. On that day Eric Starling was on his way back from Benbecula and was forced to descend and return to Balivanich where he had to delay for several hours. That the conditions thwarted a pilot of his experience is an indication of their severity. We managed to carry on only by climbing out of the rain-ice.'

'One patient with whom we had an ongoing contact was a little girl from Barra who had leukaemia. We used to fly her for treatment at fairly regular intervals. We got to know her and her family. Then the treatment became more frequent. She eventually went into hospital in Glasgow and then there was the occasional trip to take her to Barra for the holidays to be with her parents. We got to know her whereabouts at any particular time and one night we had a call-out to collect her from Barra. It took the best part of a day to get her off because of the state of the tide. A few weeks later a crew were called to operate a coffin charter to take her home. We were all deeply affected by that because it was as if we were part of that little girl's life.'

'On a lighter note, I think it was Ron Atkinson who had a very, very sick patient who was carried aboard the aeroplane in the dark. He was strapped down with much moaning and groaning, comforted and attended by the nurse. As Ron was starting up, one of the engines backfired and the exhaust caught fire. At night this is quite spectacular, to put it mildly. Ron thought he had better go into the cabin to assure the nurse and patient that everything was all right.'

'When he opened the door into the cabin he found an empty stretcher with the strap swinging off the side of it. The main cabin door was flapping gently in the breeze and in the distance were two figures, rear view, running like hell.'

'I had four engine shut-downs for a variety of reasons and I did two three-engine ferry flights. The first of these was off the beach at Barra with the tide coming in so that we hit the water before we became airborne. It took ages for us to get back to Glasgow where we were still white in the face when we reported to the Ops Room.'

'Gestures of kindness are always remembered and one of these was at Campbeltown on an ambulance flight. The wind was about 40 knots. We got the patient on board but we couldn't get one of the engines to start. The firemen held umbrellas over us as best they could as I went under the cowlings and I found I was actually tipping water out of the HT leads to the plugs. At that point we had to give up and call for an engineering flight from Glasgow.'

'The patient was taken off and, while we were awaiting the engineering flight, the Air Force let us use a very large hangar. As we taxied in my co-pilot reminded me about various rules and regulations about taxying in hangars. But we weren't going to hit anything. We shut down the engines and we were going to wait there for the engineering flight.'

'At this point the Station Superintendent, Jimmy Sheal, said, "Come on lads. Back to my place." We went back to his house to be greeted by his wife saying, "Take your clothes off. Here are some dressing gowns." We had been soaked and cold but we were now having a hot shower, followed by soup, and by the time we heard our engineering flight, which would also take the patient away, our clothing had been dried.'

'We had one night-stop on Barra when we had to get the aircraft off the beach to prevent the salt water from reaching it when the tide came in. I was taxying up the causeway on the inboard engines when the First Officer signalled me to stop while he moved the outboard propellers to horizontal to clear the sand dunes. The Heron was moored there by putting a ladder against the back of it to make sure the tail didn't tip. We made inspections during the night to ensure that the sheep weren't eating the fabric off the flying control surfaces.'

'On the occasion of my last landing at Tiree the wind was 60 knots, gusting 80. The Heron stalled at 50 knots so I thought, "There could well be problems here." I did a part flap landing on One Eight and as I came to the intersection of the runways, the fire engines were there. They drove in front of the wings to break the lift. We just sat there and virtually flew the aeroplane while they got the ambulance patient on board and then, on my signal, the fire engines drew back, I opened the throttles and we just went up vertically.'

'Some of our ambulance flights were booked in advance for the routine moving of a patient. I was doing one of these from Sumburgh to Aberdeen and in the area at the time was the recently appointed CAA flight operations inspector, Captain Fawshawe. I had met him previously when he had been our flight ops inspector on the Trident. He was a very senior pilot and I was a very new captain.'

'We went off together to Sumburgh and did the usual approach on to Three Three. I forget what the wind was, but it was extremely strong. Having made the turn and coming in over Three Three, a very large hand grabbed the aeroplane and shook it all over the place. It was clearly out of the question to attempt to land from it so round we went. To keep the runway in sight I elected to do a left hand circuit. Going down from Runway Three Three at Sumburgh we must have hit a rotor off Fitful Head because at one stage, with full left aileron applied, I had forty-five degrees of bank to the right.'

'We soon recovered and I glanced back and smiled at Captain Fawshawe who had no place to sit other than the front row of passenger seats. His knuckles were white and he was grasping the seat rest. It must have been quite frightening for him, as a very experienced pilot, not to have a set of controls available to him under those circumstances.'

Viv Gunton flew his last Heron service on 24th January 1973, a few months before the type was retired from BEA service, and he undertook an estimated 134 ambulance flights. He is now a Corcorde Captain, flying the rich and famous, and captains of industry, across the Atlantic. 'It is very difficult to decide which is more rewarding, flying at Mach 2 across the Atlantic, or serving communities on a very personal level, providing the community need that the Scottish Air Ambulance Service provided.' It is certainly a total contrast.

Lighting the Skies of Orkney

C APTAIN ANDY ALSOP is no stranger to adventurous flying, his career having taken him to the Falkland Islands where he helped develop inter-island air services and where he now flies for the British Antarctic Survey during the Austral summer.

Before that Andy was one of that select breed of Loganair pilots who earned their place in Orcadian folklore as they once again 're-pioneered' Orkney inter-island air travel, just as Edmund Fresson had done in the 1930s. It was in this role that Andy Alsop found himself in the Guinness Book of Records for flying the world's shortest scheduled flight, from Westray to Papa Westray.

Captain Alsop claims that for anecdotes he is a bit of a 'dead loss', most of the memorable events being unprintable. He limits himself to a couple of what he says are the more 'bland' ones!

'The first concerns what we claimed at the time to be a speed record for an ambulance flight. It must have been about 1977, and I was sitting in the Loganair office at Kirkwall Airport chatting to two of our regular passengers. They were both professors of medicine from Scottish universities, involved in research into multiple sclerosis, a disease particularly prevalent in Orkney. Outside the window was one of our Islanders with a stretcher already fitted. It had returned to Kirkwall from an ambulance flight to one of Orkney's North Isles about half-an-hour before, and the cabin had not yet been reconfigured for the carriage of passengers.'

'The telephone rang. The doctor on Hoy wanted a patient flown in from the airstrip at Longhope as soon as possible. Now, normally there would be a pause of ten to fifteen minutes whilst a nurse or doctor travelled out from Balfour Hospital in Kirkwall to the airport to fly in the aircraft to collect the patient. During this time the stretcher and whatever other medical equipment might be required would be fitted.'

'On this occasion there was no delay. The two professors thought it a huge joke to be invited along to act as nurses, and we were airborne within two minutes of receiving the call. The flight to Longhope took just about the normal seven minutes. As we touched down, the Hoy doctor drove up with the patient who was loaded into the aircraft in a most expeditious manner. The Islander landed back at Kirkwall Airport just a few seconds under twenty minutes from receiving the original call. The road ambulance to convey the patient to the Balfour Hospital had just reached the airport!'

'At the time we surmised that this must have been our fastest ever response. Certainly it was the most "top heavy" ambulance flight, medically speaking!'

'The second story goes back to the very early years of Loganair's operation in Orkney (begun in 1967). We had been flying to Orkney's North Isles for perhaps two or three years. It had become routine for us to fly out in the middle of the night, in poor visibility, with a low cloud base, to land on a sloping field covered with mud and cow dung with the aid of just a few paraffin flares.'

'I used to think we made it all look so easy, and that the pilots were not treated with the deference which I felt we richly deserved!'

'On this particular occasion the nurse was sitting up front with me as we flew out to collect a patient from the island of Westray. She was telling me how much harder such a flight must have been in "the old days", before the invention of radar and modern navigational beacons, etc. I tried, tactfully, to point out to her that there was no radar coverage in the north of Scotland, and that at the height at which we were necessarily flying we could not receive any assistance from radio aids. It was just dead reckoning as we flew through the dark winter's night at 500 feet in and out of quite heavy snow showers. She remained unconvinced.'

'The aircraft lights were turned down very, very low so that my eyes were accommodated for picking up the first glim flicker of the airstrip's gooseneck flares. (At that time, mains electricity had not reached Orkney's outer isles, and as no one normally ran domestic generators at 2.00am, everything below was totally black. Elsewhere in Britain there are always odd lights left on here and there to lend perspective.)'

'On the windscreen I detected the incipient signs of St Elmo's Fire, a phenomenon familiar to mariners for many years but not as commonly seen by aviators. Snow pellets falling through cold dry air were striking the perspex windscreen, causing a build-up of static electrical charge. The first visual signs, a faint dancing glow on the windscreen, had not been spotted by the nurse, who apparently remained convinced that we were still proceeding as a result of some unspecified form of automation.'

'More to reassure myself than for the nurse's benefit, I said that we were nearly there. "There", she triumphed, as she searched the unrelieved blackness. "You can't possibly know where an invisible airstrip is without navigation aids." "Oh yes, I do", I said, "it's just over there", stabbing my forefinger at the far side of her windscreen.'

'From past experience in similar atmospheric conditions, I was expecting a small spark to jump from my finger to the perspex. I hoped it might impress her! I was totally unprepared for the "bolt of lightning" which jumped in spectacular fashion, and very painfully, across the gap. The runway flares appeared right on cue, in line with the flash. The whole episode certainly impressed me!'

'The nurse never said a thing, but word must have got around. From that night on we Orkney pilots, though still not regarded as deities, were always treated with fitting reverence by the nurses.'

Lobster for Dinner

E LISABETH DOUGLAS flew as an air ambulance nurse, while based at the Southern General Hospital as a midwife, between 1967 and 1972. Elisabeth remembers her introduction to each flight by her arrival in a large room at Glasgow Airport.

'I was never quite sure what happened there, but it was always filled with cheery men and I would be plied with cups of coffee until our flight was ready to depart. Many nurses who started off enthusiastically fell by the wayside after the first flight because the Heron wasn't a terribly comfortable plane to fly in, especially if the weather was bad and there was turbulence. The aircraft wasn't pressurised, sometimes it was cold inside and sometimes it was hot. It could be quite frightening if you were flying very low in bad weather. The stretcher was extremely hard and the patients were very uncomplaining. Some of the long flights must have been very uncomfortable for them, especially when they had painful injuries.'

'Islay was the destination I felt least at ease with. There was no runway lighting other than flares. In bad weather I would peer desperately in the dark to see the runway until it appeared dimly down below. The flares were not very bright. I think my fear of Islay was heightened because one of the planes was named after Sister Jean Kennedy who lost her life on a flight to the island.'

'It is a very special experience landing on the beach at Barra. In the late spring the whole of the north end of the island is covered with primroses and it was quite idyllic sitting on the edge of the beach while waiting for the patient to arrive. But I also remember Barra for one of my worst flights. It was a winter's afternoon and I was to collect a small baby who had pneumonia. We had to fly low over the sea with tremendous turbulence all the way and I was extremely sick. When we arrived at Barra, the child, who lived on Vatersay, had not arrived because of the bad weather conditions. We had to wait for more than an hour and by the time the child arrived it was dark and the tide had turned. The captain was becoming rather agitated and a lorry took off to the water mark, turned round and shone its lights towards us.'

'The captain remarked that if we were still on the beach when we reached the lights, it was time to worry. We took off safely but we had the most horrendous journey back to Glasgow. The baby was extremely ill. As we approached Glasgow Airport the captain said that he might be unable to land because of strong cross winds. We watched a Trident go in to land and saw it overshoot the runway. We attempted it ourselves but were unable to land and had to fly on to Prestwick. Unfortunately, even with a police escort to Ayr Hospital, the baby died shortly afterwards.'

'Another call took us to Sumburgh to collect a fisherman with badly injured legs. It turned out that he was a Russian seaman. The captain of the vessel brought him to the airport and handed him over to us. It was obvious that the man was absolutely terrified. He could speak no English and seemed of the belief that he was going to be abducted into the unknown and never see his beloved Russia again. He wept copiously in the plane, clutching his passport and a small leather bag. He refused to give them up and he refused anything for pain.'

'I always admired the flexibility of the air ambulance service. I once had to take a lady, suffering from terminal cancer, from Inverness to her home in Exeter. At Inverness her doctor handed me a package which he said contained morphine. A short time after we had taken off, the patient started to complain of pain and I opened the package to discover that it was an old-fashioned type of morphine in tablet form which required to be dissolved in a metal teaspoon of sterile water over a flame. Once it had dissolved you then drew it up and gave it as an injection.'

'Although I had sterile water in my case, we had no metal teaspoons and nobody smoked, so therefore there were no matches. I explained my dilemma to the captain. He immediately called Manchester Airport by radio. We diverted and there, waiting at the terminal, was the airport nurse with a proper ampule of morphine.'

'For maternity cases we also provided the Flying Squad service. This involved going to mothers who had complications, either in labour or after they had delivered. On these flights doctors from the Maternity Unit went with us. If the placenta had been retained by the mother, the squad included a senior doctor and a senior anaesthetist. If it was a patient who was haemorrhaging, the team would include a senior doctor and a junior doctor. We took a large box containing everything that we would need to remove the placenta under general anaesthetic, and also all the equipment that we needed to transfuse the patient, usually plasma and other intravenous fluids.'

'I did three Flying Squad flights and these were all at night. Upon reaching the island we were taken by ambulance to the hospital where the patient was made fit to fly. We nearly always brought the patients back with us although occasionally they were fit enough to be left. The plane would therefore have to wait up to three or four hours until the patient was fit enough to travel. On two flights that I did, the patients arrived in Glasgow fitter than the doctors as in each case the doctors suffered from air sickness.'

'On one occasion we arrived over Glasgow in very thick fog and we circled for some time. In this instance the mother was not very well at all. We thought that we might have to divert to Prestwick when we saw a small hole in the cloud. The captain dived through it to effect a safe landing. A few days later the registrar, who had been on the flight, told me that he had received a letter from the captain saying that he was in some trouble with the authorities for "landing in unacceptably dangerous conditions". The registrar was able to tell the authorities that the patient's condition warranted such a landing. The explanation must have been accepted because the following flight I did was also under his command.'

'Once, during a shipping strike, I went on a Viscount to Shetland to pick up twenty patients who were requiring treatment at Aberdeen. Many of the patients were psychiatric cases so a psychiatric nurse was also in attendance. There were no stretcher cases and the flight was uneventful so the two of us coped with this unusually large assignment.'

'At Stornoway we had to collect a man who had fallen from a roof, fracturing his spine. He had been placed on a larger-than-average door. The Heron was of no use because the door would not go in. We were therefore using a Viscount and upon arrival at Stornoway Airport it took ten men to manoeuvre the patient up the steps of the plane. Several seats had been removed and the door was placed on the floor.'

'I could never understand why, but on arrival at Glasgow Airport they were totally unable to extract the door. It took about an hour and about thirty men to detach a panel and remove the patient.'

'While I was flying with the air ambulance service, Loganair started to do flights. These I did not enjoy. I found the aircraft to be very small and cramped and the pilot was aware of the slightest movement that might be made. There was very little space between the nurse and patient.' *

'But I do remember one wonderful flight with Loganair. We flew to Coll on a glorious evening to pick up a little girl with a broken leg. We flew between Islay and Jura, and passed low over Fingal's Cave. When we arrived at Coll, the pilot was presented with an enormous fresh lobster. The following day I received a message that there was a package for me. I went to the office to find he had asked his wife to cook the lobster for me and had sent it up to the hospital. It was an extremely nice and kind thing to do and a group of us had a wonderful party that night.'

* This was the Piper Aztec used by Loganair on its first air ambulance flights until the Britten-Norman Islander went into service.

Island Pilot

*W*HILE THE earlier account of Alan Whitfield's ambulance flight to Unst on a stormy night in 1972 illustrates how, on that occasion, he had been aided by the most advanced communications technology, a nocturnal mission from Sumburgh to Fair Isle the following year had to rely upon more rudimentary assistance.

'The ringing of the telephone dragged me from sleep and as I walked to the front hall to answer it I was aware of an unexplained sense of unease. "Halloa, Alan! Ian here. There is a problem on Fair Isle. Can we get over there as soon as possible?"

'As I reached for the air ambulance pad to record the details, I realised the cause of my unease. The Sumburgh fog horn was blowing! Looking out of the window I could see right across the airfield but the base of the cloud was very low. The lighthouse at Sumburgh is about 300 feet up and it was obviously in cloud. "It's not very good, Ian. How important is it that we go now?" "Very", came the reply. "Roger. I'll call you right back."

'Next, I called Stuart Thompson on Fair Isle. It being a small community, he already was aware of the emergency and had checked outside. "The North Light is blowing, but not the South. And I can see well to the south of the island." This confirmed my assessment of the situation. The north lighthouse is high up on the cliffs whilst the south one is at sea level. This suggested a cloud base of about 250 feet. The airstrip on Fair Isle is about 400 feet up. It was going to be tricky!'

'There was a lot more phoning to do. To the doctor to tell him I would have a go, to the air traffic controller to open up the airfield, to the Aberdeen Met Office to check on diversion airfields in case the weather in Shetland closed in completely, and finally to Stuart on Fair Isle to give him an ETA and tell him how I wanted the old-fashioned paraffin flares positioned.'

'In the days before the oil boom hit Shetland everyone lent a hand. By the time I reached the airfield, the aircraft was fuelled, one of the firemen was helping to fit the stretcher, and all was ready to go.'

'My logbook shows that twenty-eight minutes later the doctor and I were airborne. At 150 feet I found that the aircraft was just clear of the cloud and so I set course for the island. After about five minutes, fog right down to the sea forced me to climb, and at 450 feet we emerged into bright moonlight with the fog on a milky sea beneath. The visibility was good above the cloud and we could see clearly the top of Ward Hill on Fair Isle.'

'As we passed over the island the gooseneck flares were just visible through the cloud. Turning left, I started an approach, only to lose sight of everything as I entered the fog, forcing a climb back up into the moonlight. This clearly would not do and, as I had no contact with Fair Isle, I was entirely on my own. I called the controller at Sumburgh who telephoned Fair Isle and learned that it was still clear beneath the cloud to the south.'

'With this in mind, I positioned the aircraft to the south and began a very cautious descent through the cloud layer, finally sighting the sea at about 200 feet with the lighthouse clearly visible to the north. Returning towards the island, I turned right to follow the shore line, keeping it about 400 yards off my port wing. The Sheep Rock came into sight, then the Bird Observatory and, as I flew parallel to the coast, I could just see the glow of the goosenecks at the end of the strip.'

'Slowing the aircraft, I put down some flap and, lining up with the edge of a cliff which is off the end of the strip, I started an approach. As I progressed, I realised that I would enter the cloud as I climbed up the hillside towards the strip. My only chance would depend on me catching a glimpse of the first flares before I had to put on full power and climb away to a safe height. I continued the approach, watching out for a small walled enclosure, known in Shetland as a "planticrub", a place used to raise cabbage plants and which I knew was about 100 yards before the strip. I decided that, if I lost sight of that before seeing the flares, I would have to overshoot.'

'I reached the planticrub and started to open the throttles, at the same instant seeing the glow of the first flare. Selecting full flap, I closed the throttles and slammed the aircraft onto the strip, standing on the brakes as soon as it touched. When we had stopped, I taxied over to where the vehicles were awaiting us and, as the doctor was driven off down to the patient, I sat in a state of exhilarated relief at being on the ground.'

'By the time the doctor returned with the patient, the fog had closed in totally and visibility was down to a few yards. I was able to talk to Sumburgh on the radio and was told that conditions there were unchanged so, taxying to the west end of the strip, I made a blind take-off out over the sea. The return to Sumburgh was fairly routine and soon the patient was on her way to hospital while I returned home to relax over a cup of tea.'

'Of all the hundreds of ambulance flights that I carried out during my career, this is the one which sticks most in my memory and about which I still wake up sometimes in the night and give a shudder.'

A Weight off the Mind

NURSE JUNE NEIL had a winter introduction to the air ambulance and to Loganair's Islander aircraft when she first took to the air at the close of 1978.

'Despite its lightweight appearance, the wee Islander would stand up to anything, it seemed. On more than one occasion we landed on a snow-covered runway and gaily slithered to a halt, not always facing the right direction! On my first trip to Barra it wasn't the weather that was the problem, it was the sea. The tide wasn't quite full out and, when we landed, the wheels sent sea spray everywhere as again we slithered and slid to a halt. I must have looked a sight as I leapt out of the plane, cloak flapping from my shoulders, trying to avoid getting my feet wet.'

'One flight was from Glasgow to Shetland to take a young woman with suspected meningitis to Aberdeen Royal Infirmary. The flight took approximately two-and-a-half hours and usually meant a stopover at Wick or Aberdeen for fuel. After a few such flights, and especially on dark winter afternoons, the journey could be quite monotonous. The weather was pretty foul outside on this particular day, a mixture of rain, sleet, hail and snow with a bit of turbulence. However it didn't stop me from snuggling into my cloak and dozing off in the passenger seat behind the pilot.'

'Alas, my nap was interrupted as the plane approached Sumburgh. The change in the engine noise first alerted me, accompanied by some vigorous shaking of the aircraft. I leaned forward

to look at the approaching lights of the runway — we seemed to be a little "off-side".
"Not to worry," I thought, as the pilot just glanced back at me with that "everything's under control" smile.'

'But I couldn't help noticing the forceful movements of his hand at the controls. At the same time the engine noise changed from a continuous whine to an intermittent judder. I quickly looked out of the left window and could see, faintly, that the propeller was stopping and starting, stopping and starting. We were leaning to one side yet still approaching the runway. Then, with what felt like an almighty jolt, the engine resumed its continuous whine, the plane evened out and at last we were on the runway.'

'I later learned what had happened. Apparently the weather had been so cold that ice particles had started to clog up one engine, causing the propellers to, well, "judder". Thankfully the flight to Aberdeen with the patient on board was smoother and uneventful. The pilot remained his usual unruffled self and described the flight as being "a bit turbulent but otherwise fine."'

'There were times where we might gain 24-48 hours notice of a flight. On one such occasion the information was relayed that the patient would be a man who had sustained fractured verterbrae of the cervical spine (i.e., a broken neck), following a road traffic accident. Having been stabilised at Raigmore Hospital, Inverness, he was to be transferred to Dundee Royal Infirmary by air ambulance. The flight would require two nurses as he was in a special spinal frame.'

'It paid to use such advance warning to check out any special equipment or appliances which might accompany the patient. I went to the Southern General's Accident & Orthopaedic Ward the evening before the flight and was kindly "brushed up" on spinal frames by the staff. The frame included a "D-bar", a D-shaped device which was used to help turn the frame and hence the patient. It also could be removed — which was just as well.'

'The other nurse and I enjoyed a pleasant flight to Dalcross Airport, Inverness. We were met by a doctor in front of the ambulance. He explained that not only was the patient on a spinal frame, but also he had several pounds of traction attached to his skull! This meant two things. One, the weights would have to be kept still and not be permitted to swing to and fro and, two, if the patient needed to be sick, the plane would have to flip on its side in mid-air as he couldn't be moved onto his side. Why couldn't we use the D-bar to turn him? Because it had to be removed to allow the frame to fit into the plane!'

'So there we were, taking it in turns to kneel on the floor and hold the weights still throughout the whole flight. Luckily the patient didn't feel sick.'

'Our troubles weren't over when we landed alongside the River Tay at Dundee. We had managed (just) to get patient and frame into the plane, but we couldn't get him out. The ambulance men and ground staff ended up completely removing the rear door from the plane and slowly but surely eased the patient out with me steadying those weights. Despite all this the poor man thanked us for a smooth entertaining journey and expected to make a full recovery which, I believe, he did.'

'There were times when more than one request for an air ambulance would come in at the same time. My first unaccompanied flight (i.e., without another nurse) was to Jura. The information given to me was that I would be picking up an eight-year-old male with a suspected fractured leg.'

'I was excited as well as a little apprehensive as we took off on a crisp sunny afternoon. The scenery was beautiful and I looked out eagerly for the runway. Well, the runway was a field and boy, was the landing bumpy.'

'We were met by a small crowd of islanders and the local G.P. The patient was still in the ambulance sheltering from the breeze. I looked in to say "hello" and introduce myself. However, my "eight-year-old male, suspected fractured leg" turned out to be a 69-year-old lady with burns to her arm. Obviously I had been given the other air ambulance's information. I wonder what its nurse thought on her arrival!'

Born on a Plane

*J*ONATHAN AYRES from Port Ellen, Islay, does not remember much about his first flight. That is understandable since he wasn't even on the passenger list when Britten Norman Islander G-BFCX *E L Gandar Dower* took off for Glasgow in darkness from Glenegedale Airport in the early hours of 6th January 1982.

His mother was en route to Glasgow to give birth to Jonathan. But Jonathan was not about to hang about until his mother was safely delivered to the hospital. Instead he weighed into the world at a healthy 8lb 13oz, while the Islander was still high above Renfrewshire on approach to Glasgow, to join a growing list of babies to be born in the air since Loganair began air ambulance flying in 1967.

From Day One, Jonathan was set to be a young celebrity because of an unusually appropriate surname and a little foresight by his parents. The customary silver quaich, presented by Loganair to inflight babies as a unique keepsake, reads:

Jonathan Philip Logan Ayres
born 6th January 1982
at 0509 hours
above Houston, Renfrewshire
at a height of 2,000 feet
on Loganair aircraft G-BFCX
Captain D Dyer

When Loganair celebrated its 25th anniversary in 1987, Jonathan was a guest of the airline for a special visit to Glasgow, to celebrate an anniversary of his own.

At the age of eleven Jonathan still vividly recalled that occasion. 'When it was Loganair's 25 years in service my Mum, Dad, and myself were flown out to Glasgow for my 5th birthday. We had lunch at Glasgow Airport. I had a lovely birthday cake and Mr Scott Grier gave me a Lego airport set and I got to sit in the air ambulance I was born in.' Scott Grier remembers his young guest who liked to introduce in himself as 'Jonathan Ayres — born on a plane.'

When a video documentary of the air ambulance service was being prepared, the makers visited Jonathan at his school on Islay to include him in their filming sequences. When nine, Jonathan was on camera again on the children's television programme *Ghost Train*. He was one of several children selected to go to Newcastle-upon-Tyne to tell of an unusual experience. Appropriately, Jonathan's interview was recorded in an aircraft above the city.

When we spoke, Jonathan had just started his secondary education at Islay High School to which he travels ten miles by bus each day. At weekends he goes to Machrie Golf Course for golfing lessons. To work off his surplus energy he plays the drums and was looking forward to a trip to Glasgow to play football with the Port Ellen Boys Club against a team from Maryhill.

Jonathan has a younger sister, Helen, and younger brother, Benjamin, both also being born in Glasgow after their mother had been flown by air ambulance from Islay.

It is a normal routine now for expectant mothers to be flown from the Scottish islands to give birth in the security of the specialist maternity units of mainland hospitals. Mrs Ayres's recollection of Jonathan's birth on the aircraft is faint but Captain David Dyer, who was at the controls, remembers it vividly.

'I had had a birth on board an air ambulance flight from Campbeltown the previous night. That night had been extremely rough and the midwife was struggling to cope with air sickness when the patient started to give birth. Normally I would have remained in the air at this stage but it was so wild I brought the aircraft down, slapped it on to the runway, and kept it there until the birth had been completed. The air traffic controllers gave a cheer over the radio when I announced the arrival of a baby girl.'

'And here only 24 hours later was the same midwife telling me that it was about to happen again. By contrast, it was a clear still night with the moon reflecting off the snow. Margaret Ayres was propped up in the cabin behind my seat and I could feel the back of it being pushed as she laboured. Since we were going to have to circle until the birth was completed I asked her if she would like to have her baby over Greenock, Houston or Largs. Margaret chose Houston and that is where Jonathan was born.'

Margaret Ayres recalls that Helen's birth went without a hitch. But it was the birth of Benjamin that will always remain vividly in her mind. 'Serious complications set in and the air ambulance had to be called urgently. Had it not been for the speed at which I was conveyed to hospital, both myself and Benjamin would not have survived. The days when the islands did not have the air ambulance are still remembered and I will always be grateful that it was there when I needed it so desperately.'

North-west by West

D ESPITE THE major contribution by men to the nursing profession, the perception of the nurse as a solely female role is still widely, and erroneously, held. It is easy therefore to be guilty of the same presumption when envisaging air ambulance nurses. This of course is grossly inaccurate because male nurses have played a highly significant role alongside their female counterparts, and indeed their presence has been considered essential when it has been necessary to transport psychiatric patients.

John West flew '53 short of 500 flights' from his base at Glasgow's Southern General Hospital between 1982 and 1988. A big gentle man with a relaxed disposition, he is undoubtedly one of the unsung heroes of the band of male air ambulance nurses.

His very first flight was as a second nurse with a psychiatric case. 'I'd thought about doing it for some time but didn't know how I would take to it. Then I was asked to go on this flight and I found myself enjoying it. Most of my subsequent flying tended to be with general cases as there were often psychiatric nurses on standby, but I would quite often accompany psychi' cases as a second.'

'One case we refused to take. We flew to one of the Shetland islands to transfer a patient from the cottage hospital to Lerwick. The patient was a bit violent but we had assumed that he would be sedated. The consultant was unwilling to sedate him, but considering his history and the pilot's concern for the safety of the aircraft, the staff, and the patient himself, both I and the other charge nurse decided it would be better that he remained where he was. The last I heard was that the patient was to go to Lerwick the next day by scheduled flight, but whether he did, sedated or otherwise, I never heard.'

'The air ambulance pilot is responsible for his aircraft, but the patient is the responsibility of the nurse from the moment he is put on the plane until he is handed over to the receiving team if an ambulance is meeting us at the arrival airport. The exception was at Glasgow where we accompanied the patient in the road ambulance to the receiving hospital and only then was the responsibility for the patient passed on.'

'I had one instance where there was an elderly lady coming down to Glasgow from the islands. On this occasion I had a staff nurse with me as an observer. The patient was very frail and we had to give her oxygen. As soon as the plane took off she started to decline and her condition deteriorated. I had to decide if she would make it to Glasgow or if we should turn back. Such situations could be quite upsetting but the decision had to be mine. In this case I decided that it would be better to turn back.'

'Another time I uplifted an elderly man from Shetland, reluctantly, as I doubted if he would benefit from the air journey because he was so weak. While flying to Glasgow we were instructed to divert urgently to Barra to collect an injured child accompanied by his parents. While continuing on from Barra to Glasgow the elderly Shetlander then slipped away from us. But we could not let the child and his parents know of this development as it would undoubtedly have further distressed them. We had to carry on "nursing" the dead man so as to sustain an impression of normality on board.'

'On another occasion, late at night, I had a wee boy to be taken from Campbeltown to the Sick Children's Hospital in Glasgow. That night we saw the northern lights. It was the first time for me, but for that wee boy it was sheer joy. I had to sit him up to look out of the window and I could see the pleasure light up his eyes. These little things stick in the memory, and of course such distractions relax the patient who is filled with anxieties.

Elderly ladies in particular, who may never have flown before, were often very frightened and even just holding a hand and having a chat could have a great calming effect.'

'Occasionally I would accompany liver, heart, or lung transplant patients to hospitals such as Harefield. Improvisation was sometimes required, such as with a lung transplant patient who required a continuous supply of oxygen. One cylinder of oxygen was not enough and I had to get three cylinders and rig them together with needles and plaster to ensure that there was no break in the flow.'

'Several times I accompanied transplant patients through London with sirens screaming while the plane waited until the transfer to the hospital had been completed. There would usually also be a doctor in attendance and one night we arrived at the hospital to be given a message that the aircraft had had to go back without us. We had landed at an RAF field and the aircraft had to be off the ground by 8.00pm when the airfield would close for the night. We were advised to proceed to Stansted Airport where we could take a mail plane home at 2.00am. The seats had all been removed from this aircraft and the doctor sat up front with the pilot while I had to go in the back with the mail sacks.'

'Air ambulance duty brought good times and bad times. Coming into Inverness one winter's night, we had the option either of circling while the runway was defrosted or of coming straight in. I decided that we should go straight in because the patient was a serious burns case. It was fascinating to land under these circumstances. But we had to wait for an hour-and-a-half before we could take off again. On another occasion we landed at Barra to collect a patient as the tide was coming in. While still on the beach we received a message that a second patient was coming and that we should hang on a bit longer. We took off in four inches of water and sand. Interesting for us, but less so for the patient!'

Don't Let the Pain go Away

*T*HE NURSES and pilots who ferry patients to hospital during a medical emergency can often be in the thick of any drama that might surround the event. But once they have completed the flight and the patient is delivered into the care of the receiving hospital, their roles have reached their conclusions. Any subsequent news of a patient's progress will rarely filter back to the air crew. But the gratitude of patients lingers long after their discharge from hospital and return to good health.

Many flights are routine and undramatic from an operational perspective, although the emotions being experienced by the patient will frequently be very different. Such was the case on 7th February 1984 when the Reverend John Cormack of Campbeltown, suffering from a hip fracture, was flown to Glasgow. Ten years later his praise was undiminished for Nurse Alison Boyd of Paisley, as well as for the pilot, 'a young man with long fairish hair', and for the ambulance men at both ends who assisted with his stretcher.

Ian Purvis of Clachan, a Kintyre village that looks out across the Sound of Jura to Gigha and Islay, is equally filled with admiration for the people who came out of the eye of the hurricane to his aid on a winter's night in 1989. But his transfer to hospital over the same air route faced the full onslaught of the natural elements.

'It was shortly after midnight on 22nd March when I awoke with very severe stomach pains and vomiting. My wife did her best with hot bottles, etc., but after about an hour she rang our G.P., Dr Jim Graham at Muasdale, ten miles away.'

'There were gale force winds and frequent showers of hail and sleet. However he came out and, after examining me, he gave me an injection. He also made the necessary arrangements for the air ambulance and for the local ambulance to take me the 25 miles to Machrihanish.'

'After the injection the pain became less acute and Dr Graham left at about 3.00am. The ambulance came at about 4.00am and we skidded our way to the airfield where the little plane was sitting on the snow-covered, wind-swept runway.'

'By this time the pain had about gone and I felt a bit of a fraud. However, we flew to Glasgow Airport where an ambulance was waiting to take me to the Southern General Hospital. We arrived there at about 6.00am and people went into action immediately with scanners, etc.'

'I felt that the National Health Service was marvellous. On a really wild night, on my behalf, our G.P. had battled ten miles each way, two ambulance men had battled 25 miles each way, and the pilot and nurse had flown through terrible conditions from Glasgow to Machrihanish and back with me. Two more ambulance men had driven in slightly better conditions to the Southern General Hospital.'

'The pain did return during the first night in hospital which made me feel less guilty. During the next few days I was given an extensive investigation but nothing was ever found.'

'Upon my return home I wrote a letter to *The Herald* expressing my admiration for all the dedicated people involved. But it was not published.'

A Rogue Engine and a Rogue Patient

CAPTAIN BEN BAMBER is now a Training Captain with Manx Airlines. He joined Loganair in 1988 as a Twin Otter pilot with a previous background of fixed-wing and helicopter flying in the Fleet Air Arm and private helicopter companies.

'In a career that has included the drama of flying-in troops and firing rockets and missiles, spraying crops with chemicals, transporting VIPs, flying the "bucket and spade brigade" to holiday destinations, or businessmen on commuter flights, nothing has given me so much satisfaction as ambulance flying which I began with the Islander in 1989. It gives me, in common with most pilots, the feeling of having contributed something, rather than of just flying to earn a crust.'

'My first solo trip on the Islander was to Skye on 17th June 1989. The patient had suffered a terrible accident with some kind of water drilling rig. He been caught by a snapped whip-lashing cable which had amputated his hands and broken his neck. The poor chap was put in the back of the aircraft all strapped to a special framework for the journey to Glasgow. It was a nice day but the doctor came up to the front of the aircraft as we got within about

15 miles of Glasgow to ask if I could please ensure that it was an exceptionally smooth landing as any sort of a bump could terminally damage the patient.'

'The Islander has many virtues with its short field performance and ability to land on very rough strips. As a result, it has been built with a very tough undercarriage. Conversely, particularly when you are new on the aircraft, it is very difficult to land it smoothly, and there is usually a bit of a thud as you make contact with the runway.'

'To be sure of lining up for the best landing we could produce, I asked Glasgow Airport if I could have a final approach of about eight to ten miles to make absolutely sure that I was totally in the groove. Looking back with hindsight, it was way over the top, but I also remember that British Airways, British Midland, and various charter operators were being diverted and given lengthy holds and re-routes to make way for my Islander creeping down the glide-slope at 90 mph to land without incident.'

'Barra is an interesting place to land by day, but by night the landing is by widely spaced-out gooseneck flares and is very evocative of what flying must have been like in former times. Night landings at Barra are not permitted to pilots until they have made at least thirty daylight landings on the beach airstrip.'

'One call-out to Islay was for a diver. He had come up from a deep dive too quickly, causing the nitrogen to expand in his blood stream (a condition known as the "bends" and which can cause very serious injuries). To fly him to hospital meant staying at very, very low altitude, resulting in a wave-top cruise from Islay back to the mainland, following the Clyde and then actually having to climb to land at Glasgow.'

'A colleague had a similar low level flight from Orkney, having to follow the length of the Great Glen, skimming the surface of Loch Ness at zero feet.'

'Islay was the location of my most dramatic ambulance flight. The patient was an expectant mother whose pregnancy had developed some complications. It was in the middle of a fairly mediocre night. The patient was boarded and we set off again for the mainland. Just after we had taken off and before we had gone into the clouds, one of the engines started coughing and spluttering and the aircraft started yawing back and forth. Still below the cloud base, the easiest thing to do was make a quick circuit and land to investigate the problem.'

'As is usually the case, the problem refused to re-appear when we landed, and despite trying everything in the book and a few things not in the book, I could not reproduce the fault. Had this been a regular flight we would probably have waited until an engineer came out, but because this was a relatively urgent case, I elected to try again to return to Glasgow. This time we climbed into the cloud and the problem recurred worse than ever.'

'The aircraft yawed from side to side quite violently as one of the two engines cut in and out. I was contemplating whether I would have to close one of the engines down when the nurse came up to the front and very coolly and professionally asked, "Is it normal for smoke and flames to be coming out of the left-hand engine?" Time seemed to stop. I spun round but could not see the flames, just a glow at the rear of the aircraft. I told her that there was no problem at all and the aircraft could fly perfectly well on one engine, whilst at the same time trying to shut that engine down as quickly as possible.'

'We climbed on through the cloud on the one remaining good engine. Because of the weather at Islay and the condition of the patient I decided to continue. This was shortly after the crash of a British Midland Boeing 737 at Kegworth where indications suggested that cross-wiring had resulted in the wrong engine being closed down after one engine had failed. On my first departure from Islay there had been a mix-up in the communications link and Islay had told Glasgow that I was having trouble with the right engine. When I then called them up and said that I had shut down the left engine, there was consternation and concern that I had shut down the wrong engine. I assured Glasgow that we had shut down the engine that the smoke and flames were coming from so we were reasonably confident that it was the faulty engine that we had closed down.'

'We made a landing at Tiree at about 11.30 one night, with a very small and slightly-built nurse on board to receive the patient. As we taxied in, the doctor ran out to meet us with the news that there had been a mis-diagnosis. Our information on leaving Glasgow had been that the patient was an epileptic who had had a major fit. It now transpired that the patient was suffering the after-effects of two bottles of whisky and several pints of beer. According to the doctor, what would have been a very effective treatment for the epileptic fit was a very bad treatment for extreme quantities of alcohol. The patient was now in a fighting-mad rage and he could not be sedated because of the drugs already administered.'

'The doctor was still anxious that the man be admitted for observation, partly because of the alcohol consumed and partly because of the drugs that he had subsequently been given. ''Would we still take him back?'' was the doctor's question. Seeing the doubting glances exchanged between the nurse and myself, the doctor suggested that we come and see the patient so as to reach a decision.'

'We went into the firemen's duty room where the patient was being 'held', and, as we walked in, it either sparked off or coincided with one of his violent takes. I shall never forget the sight of this six-foot-plus islander, who seemed to be nearly as broad. He had a fireman on each arm and had a policeman holding him by the neck yet he was still managing to charge across the room towards me. We ducked back out into the corridor and the patient actually escaped. He went running across the airfield and had to be recaptured by the combined efforts of the police, the fire brigade, and the doctor's assistant.'

'As you can imagine, we were not particularly keen to have him on the aircraft. However we remained for several hours while sedative was administered at half-hourly intervals. Eventually he succumbed and conked out. We stretchered him out to the Islander but the little nurse, who was about 4' 10" in high heels, was not very happy about being the only person in the back with him. It was decided to handcuff the patient to the stretcher, legs and arms, and we also took one of the policemen and one of the firemen with us, carrying truncheons for use if an emergency arose. However, the patient remained sedated throughout the flight and eventually returned to Tiree with the father and mother of all hangovers.'

Paramedic Pioneers

N ATIONWIDE AIR ambulance cover of Scotland by helicopter was launched in 1993, but the groundwork for this had been preceded by an experiment based at Dundee Airport and launched in 1989. Gerry Kelly, Robert 'Syd' Devine and Ian Golding were three of the paramedics who flew with the Dundee helicopter which was sponsored by British Telecom and its operator, Bond Helicopters Ltd.

'There were many sceptics when the helicopter service was introduced on an initial six-month experimental basis from Dundee', reflects Gerry Kelly. 'Yet many of those critics were quick to appreciate its value once they had seen it in action and we soon won the support of many who had initially doubted its effectiveness. Indeed interest developed rapidly and we often found ourselves on the ground at hospitals for an hour or more after delivery of a patient, giving demonstrations of the facilities provided on the Bölkow BO 105 to senior doctors and medical officials whose curiosity had been stimulated by our arrival.'

The role of the Dundee helicopter was primarily to handle on emergency situations, such as road accidents or injuries on the Scottish mountains. The expanded role of the helicopter service launched in 1993 still includes a vital emergency function but a portion of its work is the transporting of patients living in remote locations to hospital.

Most patients were brought to Dundee Royal Infirmary or Ninewells Hospital. There were no formal helicopter pads as is now the case at many major Scottish hospitals but both institutions were well endowed with adequate wide open space for landings. But Phil Green, the helicopter pilot, was adept at putting down in the unlikeliest of places. 'These included the approaches of the Forth Road Bridge and the deck of a lighthouse supply vessel in the Firth of Tay', recalls Ian Golding. 'One of the more difficult places was Aberfeldy where we were called to a road accident. I shall always remember Aberfeldy for its trees. There are trees everywhere. We eventually found a house with a large back garden. We landed there to the bewilderment of the lady of the house. We apologised for using her garden, attended the accident and returned with the patient. The lady still seemed to be suffering from shock as we prepared to take-off. All she said was, ''Call back in again any time you want to.''

The concept of paramedics serving the Scottish Ambulance Service was in its infancy when the helicopter service was launched. In addition to personnel being trained for this new role, supplementary training had to be undertaken for them to serve on the helicopter. Navigation was one of the further skills considered necessary for the air ambulance paramedics because visual flying was the order of the day, and the door pocket of the helicopter was always bulging with Ordnance Survey maps to aid the crew.

'But we could still encounter problems finding our way,' reflects Syd Devine. 'On one occasion we were flying in high winds and were trying to locate the scene of an accident near Auchterarder. We spotted a police car parked in a lay-by so landed behind it to ask directions. Because of the wind, they had not heard our approach and we gave them quite a shock when we appeared from nowhere at the car window.'

On another occasion Ian Golding was on a flight trying to reach the scene of an accident on the A9 trunk road in extremely poor visibility. 'We found that the best way of following the winding route through the mountains was to fly above a large articulated truck which stood out well in the mist. This was progressing well until suddenly a bridge crossing the A9 appeared from nowhere and the pilot had to take swift evasive action to avoid colliding with it. The driver of a Ford Escort on the bridge had an even bigger fright than we did.'

Ian Golding and Syd Devine were the paramedics on a flight called to assist in the search for a light aircraft that had crashed in the Borders. 'Again the weather was misty,' says Syd Devine. 'It was difficult to navigate and we were off course. Suddenly we saw the plane, its nose stuck into the side of a hill. The pilot had been 10 miles off in his estimate of his last position and everyone else was searching for him in the wrong place. It had been pure chance that we had drifted off course and accidentally found him as a result.'

'I remember Ian leaping from the side of the helicopter as it hovered close to the damaged aircraft,' recalls Syd. 'We pulled the pilot out of his aircraft and we then sent Ian running down the side of the mountain to locate a farmhouse to find out where we were so that we could radio our position. A SAR Sea King arrived and took the patient to hospital leaving us to return to our other duties. We were soaked when we climbed back into the Bölkow. We put this down to the mist and drizzle until we became aware of a strange smell. It was only then that we realised that we had been drenched with fuel leaking from the crashed aircraft.'

Leaping from the helicopter and sprinting over mountains was probably not how the paramedics envisaged their role when they were assigned to the Bölkow BO 105, even although their fitness training included 'being able to run one mile in under eight minutes'. But it happened on more than one occasion. On 14th May 1989 they were requested by the RAF's Rescue Co-ordination Centre at Pitreavie to transport the victim of a climbing accident on Ben Lawers from a mountain hut, where she was reported to have been taken by the Mountain Rescue Team, to hospital. When Gerry Kelly and Ian Golding arrived at Ben Lawers they discovered that the Mountain Rescue Team had not yet reached the injured woman. Rather than wait for what could be hours, they decided to fly to the cloud base then set off on foot with their patient-care rucksacks to where the patient lay, 800 feet below the summit of the mountain.

Working with the Search and Rescue services occurred on several occasions. The team was returning to Dundee from Kinlochrannoch, carrying a patient with a minor back injury, when they were asked to divert to Blair Atholl because of a reported drowning in Glen Tilt. The pilot made contact with SAR at Pitreavie and arrangements were made for their patient to continue by road ambulance while the air ambulance crew started to search for the victim until SAR could reach the scene.

When a climbing accident occurred on Polney Crags near Dunkeld, landing proved to be a problem. In his report on the incident Gerry Kelly described the situation, 'On arrival we flew over the scene, quickly realising that, with no landing site nearby and the poor egress from the base of the crag, the Search and Rescue services would be required to winch the casualty from the accident locus. This decision was made very quickly between aircrew and pilot. The pilot then manoeuvred close to the scene where he was able to land one skid on the hillside — which incidentally sloped at an angle of approximately 80°. However this was sufficient to allow the paramedic to exit the aircraft and render advanced life support to the casualty who had suffered back and hip injuries. The casualty, although stable, was in great pain and hypotensive. He was treated with entonox, fracture immobilisation, and an intravenous infusion. When Search and Rescue arrived he was transferred onto the Neil Robertson stretcher and winched on board. The ambulance paramedic travelled with the casualty in the Wessex to Dundee Royal Infirmary.'

The transfer of the helicopter early in 1990 from Tayside to Inverness brought an end to a short but exciting era for the city's ambulance service. But Gerry, Ian, and Syd, along with their other colleagues, take continued satisfaction from the knowledge that their work as paramedics on the *First Air* helicopter has made them modern-day pioneers.

The Yellow Budgie

*J*UST AS Jimmy Orrell was the pioneer of air ambulance flying in the 1930s, and David Barclay was the legendary ambulance captain of the 1940s, 1950s and 1960s, Phil Green of Bond Helicopters is the pioneer captain of the 'Yellow Budgies', the Bölkow BO 105D helicopters.

The Bölkow BO 105D is very much the air ambulance of the 1990s. Yet the original version first took to the air in 1967 and it has become the foremost choice for aerial medevac services in many countries, at the forefront of which is Germany, country of the helicopter's manufacture. The involvement of Scotland and of Phil Green dates from 1989 when the initial experimental service started from Riverside Airport, Dundee.

'The Dundee operation was launched in April 1989 but the preparatory work began three months earlier. In addition to the setting up of training and organisation in conjunction with Tayside Ambulance Service, this period was used to survey suitable landing sites. Eighty-eight secondary landing sites were located throughout Tayside, Fife, and the Borders, with a further thirteen sites at hospitals.'

'We moved up to Inverness for a one-month experimental period from 1st February 1990 and have operated from here ever since. We cover the northern half of Scotland with 45 secondary landing sites at our disposal — the Prestwick-based Bölkow BO 105D which covers southern Scotland has over 100 secondary landing locations.'

A large wall map in one corner of the duty room at Inverness is covered by an array of coloured pins which seem to gather in swarms around the more heavily populated areas. Red pins are particularly prominent as these mark primary landing sites being the scenes of accidents where the helicopter has required to get as close as possible. In selecting these landing sites the pilot will often have had to negotiate unforgiving terrain or to position himself close to awkwardly placed overhead cables. Most of the red pins are on main roads but there is the occasional one up a mountain, on an isolated beach, or by a river bank. The Isle of Canna, population 20, had two call-outs within a short space of time, while, thanks to the helicopter, the Isle of Muck has at last had a successful air ambulance evacuation — sixty years after Jimmy Orrell landed there in his de Havilland Dragon, only to discover that his patient had been taken away by boat. One flight not highlighted was from Hirta, largest island of the St Kilda group, because the map does not extend to this remote Atlantic outpost.

Andy Fuller explains the weighted pendulum which runs from the point on the map which marks the base at Inverness through a pulley to dangle down the frame of the chart. A quick pull of the weight extends it from the fulcrum of Inverness to the location of the next call-out, giving an instant indication of distance 'as the crow flies' and the time it will take to arrive there. Andy was the first air ambulance paramedic to be based at Inverness and has now nearly 800 missions to his credit.

Today has been a quiet day so far which is as well. There is a gale blowing outside and the radio is reporting winds ranging from 60 to 80 knots. Mike Bond, pilot on duty today, has advised the Control Desk in Aberdeen that they can take calls covering the east coast from Aberdeen up to Wick. Phil Green explains that they could operate in these conditions throughout their area in case of emergency but once the Bölkow BO 105D was over the mountains in such winds it would be pretty uncomfortable for a patient.

Instead we take a look at G-BUIB which has been wheeled behind the closed doors of the hangar. The winds rattle the giant shutters and the corrugated skin of the hangar relentlessly while the helicopter sits at peace within. Bristling with sophisticated avionics and with medi-packs stored compactly into every available space, the Bölkow looks extremely crowded for a pilot, two medical attendants, and two stretchers, but the interior layout and economical use of available space make the Bölkow eminently suitable for its air ambulance role.

The stretchers extend into what might otherwise be a baggage hold and are loaded from clam-shell doors at the rear of the aircraft. Medical treatment to stabilise a patient is generally given on the ground, but the layout means that both medical staff have access to the patient during his journey should further aid be required.

'We do not often have to carry two patients,' remarks Phil Green. 'However if a relative insists on accompanying the patient, we say they are welcome... so long as they are happy to travel while strapped into the second stretcher.'

Phil obviously feels at one with the machine. 'I should probably be flying something a bit bigger, like the Puma, but the Bölkow BO 105D is ideally suited to this job and I feel there is none better for the air ambulance role.' He is probably the most experienced Bölkow BO 105D air ambulance pilot operating in the UK, with nearly 2,000 air ambulance missions in his log book. In the same team are Mike Bond and Jeff Bond also with high hours logged on this type.

With that number of missions behind him, it is difficult for Phil Green to isolate particular instances and say they stand out more than the others. 'The birth of Mark was memorable of course,' says Phil. This is a reference to Mark Waugh, the only baby so far to be born on the Scottish Air Ambulance helicopter. Mark was ten weeks early when his mother was being rushed over the mountains in premature labour. Mark was not to be deterred and he was delivered after the helicopter made an emergency stop near Loch Riathachan. He was born in the breech position and the umbilical cord was entangled around his neck. The paramedics were Kenny MacKenzie of Inverness and Dave Haggerty of Aviemore and they took it in turn to keep tiny Mark alive until the hospital was reached.

Although road accidents are regular occurrences, there seems no limit to the variety of other ways in which people have misadventures. The list of call-outs answered by the helicopter is a litany of the bad luck of those who have subsequently become its passengers. A soldier ended up with a pellet in his eye when a youngster found him a more interesting target than those on the funfair stall that the man in khaki was supervising. A farm worker was gored by a bull which then hung around to watch the airlift of its victim. A child dragged from the rubble of a derelict house which collapsed on him, the pilot of a glider which lost contact with the thermals in spectacular fashion, and the farmer who fell foul of his mechanical potato harvester: the Yellow Budgie has been there for them all in their hour of need.

Fitness is one of the criteria for qualification as an air ambulance paramedic. One of their number was not amused when he had to scale a 150-foot rock face, only to be greeted by the injury victim with the comment that if he looked after his fitness a bit better he would not be so puffed after his climb. There's gratitude for you.

In another instance Mike Bond had to lower the helicopter into a tree-lined ravine with a swift torrent running through it. 'I was able to put one skid on the left bank of the river, where the patient lay, to let the paramedics off, but they couldn't get back on again from that position. I had to land on the opposite bank and they waded across the river. The water was absolutely freezing.' 'How do you know?' interjected Phil Green. 'Because I dipped my finger in!' was Mike's immediate reply.

'The station now operates seven days a week from 0830 until 1630, and this will extend until 1730 in the summer.' explains Phil. The wall map with its hundreds of pins is a visual picture of how the helicopter has enhanced air ambulance cover of Scotland by adding wide areas of the mainland to the communities of the islands and Kintyre peninsula who are the traditional beneficiaries of air ambulance assistance. Truly nationwide cover has arrived.

Islander in Action

I T IS Saturday 25th May 1995. I'm not a morning person but I have had to get up earlier than this. Or so I try to console myself. As luck would have it, the blue skies and sunshine of recent weeks are not favouring us with their presence today — the heavens are laden with stacks of grey cumulus, and pools of water dot the tarmac as testament to heavy rainfall throughout the night.

The scene is Glasgow Airport and I am joining Captain Dave Dyer for an air ambulance flight to Stornoway. Dave checks the weather conditions with Ops and gets a briefing on the Britten-Norman Islander BN2B G-BLNW. He is told that the aircraft had been called out at 3.00am to fly to the Orkney island of Sanday to uplift a teenager with a dislocated kneecap. One of the fuel gauges had registered empty during the return flight. A float in the tank had been misbehaving but it had been rectified by the engineers during the remaining hours of darkness.

'NW is not the regular ambulance aircraft for the Glasgow-originating flights. It is normally based at Kirkwall. The regular Glasgow-based ambulance Islander, operated by Loganair on behalf of the Scottish Ambulance Service, lies in bits in the hangar while undergoing a routine check by the engineers.

We are joined by our paramedic, resplendent in his green uniform. John has been on call for the last seven days and has already been both to Stornoway and Benbecula on four occasions during that time to accompany patients. Having become an expert at snatching precious sleep whenever the opportunity arises, he is soon slumbering in the back of the Islander.

Pre-flight checks completed, Dave awaits clearance from the tower before taxying on to Glasgow's main runway. A British Midland Boeing 737 sends up a shower of spray as it brakes heavily in order to turn-off at number 4 taxiway and permit us a swift clearance on to the main runway. The Islander needs but a few feet of it before it is airborne. A brief view of the River Clyde estuary accompanies our initial ascent and then we are into a white sea of nothingness as we are enveloped by the thick rain clouds.

The gaudily coloured pea-green Islander, which seems to be due a place of honour in an Edward Lear verse, rides the weather comfortably. We climb to 7,500 feet with the only adjustment required being an occasional de-icing of the frost that gathers on the leading edge of the wings. We have an obliging tail wind and 30 minutes out of Glasgow we catch glimpses of the mountains of Lochaber.

The cloud is soon left behind as we pass over Plockton, the township's airstrip clearly visible, and we head out to sea across The Minch to the Outer Hebrides. The radio is tuned to Stornoway which informs us that G-BIMU, the giant Sikorsky S61N Search and Rescue helicopter of HM Coastguard's Stornoway base, is heading our way. Ten minutes later we see the giant machine, a gleaming white dot in the distance, on route to the Cuillin Mountains on the Isle of Skye in search of lost climbers. As it flies beyond radio contact with Stornoway, Dave acts as a relay station to pass on a final message before it reaches the area of its search.

In the middle of the calm waters of The Minch, the Shiant Isles float like great black icebergs. These uninhabited islands were often the setting for childhood stories of marooned lighthouse keepers and of deserted ships being carried by seas that didn't know the meaning of 'calm'. The Minch can be a wild place during a storm.

But for the moment the sun is shining on the Isle of Lewis. The control tower advises us that the road ambulance delivering our patient has been delayed. Time for a cup of coffee in the airport's terminal building perhaps? We meet the crew of a Loganair Shorts 360 who are whiling away the hours between a morning newspaper delivery run from Glasgow and the afternoon passenger schedule to Benbecula. The cafeteria is just opening, and at a Hebridean pace. The road ambulance has arrived. Coffee has to be forgotten as we rush back to the Islander.

Our patient is an elderly lady with a cardiac condition and she is accompanied by her daughter. But she doesn't let her ailment get the better of her. She declines the specially fitted stretcher, and chats contentedly from a seat in the back of the Islander. 'Would we pass over her house?' she enquires. 'Where is it?', asks Dave. 'It's on the west side of the island.' our patient replies with anticipation. 'Sorry,' replies Dave. 'We don't go in that direction. That would cost you extra,' he adds mischievously.

No great drama on this ambulance run but it isn't always like that. Some patients are badly injured or have illnesses that make the flight to the specialist care of a city hospital a race against the grim reaper. Some patients are expectant mothers — Dave has lost the race with the stork on three occasions which resulted in his arrival with one more passenger than he started out with.

We curve over the terminal building as we take off from Stornoway and soon we are heading south-west towards the Isle of Skye and the mainland. We have only a few glimpses of deserted silver beaches on sparsely inhabited indentations of the West Highland coastline before we are engulfed by the rain clouds once more. A squall viciously splatters rain off the cockpit and, as we cross the highest mountain ranges, we climb from 7,500 feet to 9,500 feet to avoid turbulence. The radio crackles with messages from a Loganair Twin Otter making its approach to Glasgow on a scheduled run from the beach landing strip on the Isle of Barra. We should just land ahead of it.

Our southward journey has taken 90 minutes compared with 65 minutes northbound and we are only 7 miles from the main runway when we come out of the cloud at 1,000 feet for an ILS approach. The tower advises us to beware of surface water on the runway. We land on its vast expanse with an impertinent disregard for its miles of excess concrete. 'NW taxies direct to the Loganair hangar where an ambulance is awaiting our patient. John goes back to base to catch some more sleep while Dave dashes off to meet some of his colleagues to attend a ship-launch — Loganair pilots all seem to be shipping enthusiasts these days.

One of the hundreds of Scottish Air Ambulance flights to be flown each year has come to an uneventful and successful conclusion. Which is just how it should be.

Over by Air to Skye

O N 6TH JUNE 1935 Dr David Fyfe Anderson travelled with Northern and Scottish Airways Ltd on an air ambulance flight to the Isle of Skye. His pen recorded the event for posterity.

A youthful medico was I
When asked one day to fly to Skye
A lady gravely ill to see
And do what best for her would be.
There was no airfield there; what's more,
No doctor had flown there before.
Inside a plane I'd never been
Or at close quarters had one seen.
This was a special chartered flight
That must be made in broad daylight;
Insurance cover there was none;
I simply had the risk to run.
The pilot, engineer and I
A ten-seat plane would occupy,
With seats removed for room to make
Should I a stretcher have to take.
From Renfrew to the Misty Isle
Took only just a little while:
The many miles were swiftly spanned;
The problem then was where to land.
How many times the plane swooped low
I did not count, but this I know,
The clumps of heather were so near
My heart was in my mouth I fear.
At length we risked a landing place:
The engineer jumped out; his face
immediately showed great distress;
He shouted out, 'We're in a mess,
A bog, we must get right away,
We'll sink if any time we stay.'
My circulation almost froze;
I know not how the pilot rose,
But rise he did, came down once more
To find conditions as before,
But not so bad: they let me out
And, with a hearty, parting shout,
Instructed me to go and find
The patient whom I had in mind;
Meantime they'd search for landing ground
And would inform me when found.

Like Abraham of old, I went,
Not knowing whither, and I spent
What seemed an age, just plodding on
Until all sense of time had gone,
Through dreary bog, in weather bleak:
I now was feeling somewhat weak;
Each hand was weighted with a bag;
My energy began to sag.
How many yards or miles I walked,
And to myself in silence talked,
I cannot tell: when I beheld
A kilted man, I simply yelled,
'Can you tell me where Broadford lies?'
My fading hopes began to rise.
'Are you the doctor?' I enquired.
He answered 'No.' It then transpired
It was his wife I'd come to see,
And what a worried man was he!
He'd watched the plane's delayed descent,
Then quickly to this road-end went.
We drove along a rocky road
And came at last to his abode.
One glance at his sick darling wife
Told me if I could save her life

With me to Renfrew she must fly
Without delay, or else she'd die.
Meanwhile the questing pilot found
A solid, safer landing ground
Upon the island of Pabay,
About a mile or so away.
By ambulance we slowly drove;
On a stony track our way we wove,
While neighbours, some with tearful eyes,
Stood round about to wave Goodbyes.
We came to a derelict unused pier
And, over boulders lying near,
The stretcher was with care conveyed
And on a motor-boat was laid:
The sail to Pabay was quite brief;
We reached it safely with relief.

The conversation in the boat
Was animated, with a note
Of consternation now and then
Among these sturdy fishermen.
Now while my hearing is quite good,
No single word I understood.
The explanation came to me
Much later, over cups of tea,
When Angus gave detailed translation
Of the sea-voyage conversation.
It was in Gaelic that they chatted
And spoke as if it really mattered
That Morag should disappear
Into the dreary atmosphere.
They thought she was as good as dead
And this, in fact, is what they said: —
'How can you let your dear wife go
Off with a man you do not know
In an aeroplane that may fly on
To Cairo, Moscow, or Canton?
He is a very young man, too;
You never know what he might do!'

The patient then was put aboard
The waiting plane, and off we soared:
As we took off, torrential rain
Bespattered our small aeroplane;
Had she been drenched upon the boat,
The patient's chances were remote:
The fact which must be borne in mind
Is, Providence was very kind.

The need for fuel forced us down
At cold and rain-swept Campbeltown.
We came to Renfrew and then from there
I took my charge to nursing care
In Glasgow, where I supervised
The treatment which I had advised.
She did not, as I dreaded, die:
Weeks later, home she went to Skye
In health, without distress or strain,
But not by plane, — by railway train.

These helpful hands and willing feet
I felt much privileged to meet:
No trouble for them was too much;
I wish that there were more of such.
Team-work achieved the hoped-for cure
Which gave to all concerned joy pure.

Appendix 1
The Babies Born on Planes — A Roll of Honour

As expectant mothers have increasingly elected to give birth to their babies in hospital rather than at home, maternity cases have been a regular feature of air ambulance work since the 1930s. If a mother is anxious to have her baby in hospital with all the attendant medical expertise and equipment, it therefore follows that foregoing that objective, to replace it with the confined conditions of the cabin of a small aircraft, is not something that is entered into with any romantic illusions. A birth before arrival at hospital is not an event which is planned and it is avoided if at all possible. If a mother is in an advanced stage of labour, the nurse and pilot are always anxious to deliver their charge on to the ground and into the labour theatre. Inevitably there have been some occasions when this has not been achieved.

Tribute is therefore paid here to the babies who entered the world via an aircraft cabin; and to their mothers, the nurses who performed the delivery under such challenging circumstances, and the pilots who had to keep a steady hand on the joy stick while it was all happening.

The following is a list of all known births occurring on ambulance aircraft in Scotland. With the exception of the McLean twins, born on an aircraft of Northern & Scottish Airways in 1938 and subsequently publicised in the press, stillborn births have been intentionally omitted. Aside from these unfortunate instances, the list is believed to be comprehensive. However the author would welcome details of any births on air ambulance aircraft in Scotland which have not been included so that any omissions might be rectified at some future opportunity.

Northern & Scottish Airways

09 May 38	Baby McLean (F)	Askernish — Renfrew
09 May 38	Baby McLean (F)	Askernish — Renfrew
		Twins — Stillborn

British European Airways

22 Nov 49	John McLellan at Stornoway Airport	Benbecula — Stornoway Rapide G-AHXZ
28 Feb 50	Lachlan Macneill Macfarlane over Scarba	Tiree — Renfrew Rapide G-AHXX
03 Apr 57	Mary Agnes MacLellan Renfrew Airport	Benbecula — Renfrew Heron G-ANXB
18 Jul 57	Alexander Ewen MacPherson Renfrew Airport	Sollas — Renfrew Heron G-ANXA
31 Jan 59	Belle Anne Macleod over Garelochhead	Barra — Renfrew Heron G-ANXA
06 Apr 60	Isabel Carmichael over Gourock	Islay — Renfrew Heron G-ANXB
04 Sep 61	Iain MacLean 5,000' over Largs	Islay — Renfrew 3lb 11oz Heron G-ANXB
01 Sep 63	Alexander Thomas Gillies Bishopton	Barra — Renfrew 5lb 7oz Heron G-ANXB
04 Feb 67	David Alexander McCallum Over Ardrossan	Campbeltown — Glasgow Heron G-ANXB
30 Sep 72	Thelma McArthur 5,000' over Isle of Bute	Islay — Glasgow Heron G-ANXA

Loganair

02	Aug	73	Katy Ferguson Leynair Devin	Stronsay — Aberdeen	
			2,000' above Kirkwall	9lb 2oz G-AWNR	
05	Jun	74	Vanessa Margaret Macaskill	Benbecula — Glasgow	
			7,500' over Mull	6lb 5oz G-AXVR	
01	Dec	76	Margo Spence	Unst — Lerwick	
			2,000' above Whalsay	5lb 12½oz G-AXVR	
25	Jul	79	Angela Aileen Stevens	Shetland — Aberdeen	
			50 miles east of Wick	G-BDVW	
27	Mar	80	Angela Lydia Farrell	Islay — Glasgow	
			4,000' above Largs	G-BEEG	
03	Jul	81	Donald MacFie Swanson	Islay — Glasgow	
			7,000' above Skipness, Argyll	G-BANL	
05	Oct	81	Anthony Stephen Brocklebank	Shetland — Aberdeen	
			4,000' above Pentland Firth	2lb 10oz G-BFCX	
04	Jan	82	Anne Liese Harding	Lerwick — Aberdeen	
			2,000' 4 miles E of Fraserburgh	G-BEEG	
05	Jan	82	Sarah Jane Macdonald	Campbeltown — Glasgow	
			Glasgow Airport	6lb 2oz G-BFCX	
06	Jan	82	Jonathan Philip Logan Ayres	Islay — Glasgow	
			2,000' 4 miles W of Houston	8lb 13oz G-BFCX	
13	Aug	82	Lynsey Gray Henderson (F)	Lerwick — Aberdeen	
			10 miles N of Rattray Head	5lb 7oz G-BEEG *	
13	Aug	82	David Adrian Henderson	Lerwick — Aberdeen	
			Aberdeen Airport	5lb 14½oz G-BEEG *	
27	Jan	85	Stuart James Eunson	Lerwick — Aberdeen	
			Aberdeen Airport	7lb 6½oz G-BEEG	
05	Feb	85	Craig Martin	Campbeltown — Glasgow	
			Glasgow Airport	G-BFCX	
27	Apr	86	Amanda Lesley McAlpine	Lerwick — Aberdeen	
			45 miles NE of Aberdeen	G-BFNV	
20	Sep	87	Steven Cameron	Islay — Glasgow	
			5,500' 23 miles W of Glasgow	G-BANL	
10	Dec	89	Lisa May Kerr	Islay — Glasgow	
			Above Dunoon	G-BLNW	
27	Jan	90	Nicol William Jolly	Kirkwall — Aberdeen	
			50' over threshhold of Runway 16,	G-BLNW	
			Aberdeen Airport		
26	Sep	91	Catherine Flora McNaughton	Islay — Glasgow	
			4 miles NW of Gigha Island	G-BPCA	
26	Jul	92	Duncan Calum MacArthur McPhee	Islay — Glasgow	
			5,000' above Largs	G-BEDZ	
10	May	94	Naomi Juliet Cribb	Islay — Glasgow	
			Glasgow Airport	G-BPCA	

* Twins — born on Friday, the Thirteenth!
All Loganair births have occurred on Britten-Norman Islander aircraft.

Bond Helicopters

29	Nov	90	Mark Ian Marshall Waugh	Balmacara-Inverness
			on slopes of Meall	3lb 4oz
			Bac a' Choll Dhoire	Bölkow BO 105D G-BATC

Bristow Helicopters operating for HM Coastguard SAR

02	Apr	89	Kirsty Macleod	North Uist — Stornoway
			Over Loch Erisort	Sikorsky S-61 G-BIMU

Appendix 2

A Chronology of Six Decades
of the Scottish Air Ambulance Service

11 August	1930	Medicine flown to Islay by City of Glasgow Bombing Squadron.
19 December	1932	Midland & Scottish Air Ferries formed by John Sword.
13 April	1933	Highland Airways formed by Edmund Fresson.
14 May	1933	First air ambulance flight. Islay to Renfrew.
22 May	1933	First Outer Hebrides ambulance flight. Renfrew to Locheport, North Uist.
11 November	1933	First ambulance flights by Highland Airways.
12 January	1934	Aberdeen Airways formed by Eric Gandar Dower.
21 November	1934	Northern & Scottish Airways formed by George Nicholson.
11 January	1935	Northern & Scottish Airways' first ambulance flight — flown by Captain Charles Almond in DH Dragon G-ACFG
27 May	1935	David Barclay's first ambulance flight. Islay to Renfrew.
2 February	1936	First ambulance flight by Aberdeen Airways. South Ronaldsay to Stromness.
14 January	1937	Campbeltown Co-operative Society ambulance scheme commenced.
13 February	1937	Aberdeen Airways renamed Allied Airways (Gandar Dower) Ltd.
26 April	1937	John Hankins lands on Monach Isles to uplift lighthouse keeper's daughter, Betty McKenzie.
30 April	1937	Henry Vallance of Allied Airways lands at Esha Ness lighthouse, Shetland.
12 August	1937	Highland Airways and Northern & Scottish Airways combine to form Scottish Airways.
1 March	1938	Margaret Boyd and Jean Govan of Paisley Nurses Association contracted to provide the first regular air ambulance nurses to accompany each flight.
9 May	1938	Twins stillborn on flight from Askernish, South Uist, to Renfrew.
February	1942	First ambulance nurses supplied by Southern General Hospital, Glasgow.
1 February	1947	British European Airways takes over the services of Scottish Airways.
11 February	1948	Edmund Fresson's last ambulance flight.
5 July	1948	National Health Service established.
22 November	1949	John McLellan born in Rapide G-AHXZ upon arrival at Stornoway.
28 February	1950	First live birth in the air. Lachlan Macfarlane born over Scarba, en route to Renfrew from Tiree.
December	1952	Northern Regional Hospital Board announces plans to survey the Highlands and Islands for helicopter landing sites.
4 March	1955	First Heron ambulance flight. Benbecula to Renfrew.
28 May	1955	Last Rapide ambulance flight. Campbeltown to Renfrew.

20 February	1957	Heron G-ANXA damaged during familiarisation flight to Coll.
28 September	1957	Heron G-AOFY crashes on Islay during ambulance flight resulting the deaths of Captain Paddy Calderwood, Radio Officer Hugh McGinlay and Sister Jean Kennedy.
28 November	1958	First Silver Wings presented to air ambulance nurses.
1 February	1962	Loganair formed by Willie Logan as the aviation division of Duncan Logan Construction Co Ltd with Duncan McIntosh as Chief Pilot.
29 April	1965	David Barclay flies his last ambulance flight, from Shetland to Aberdeen, before his retirement the following day.
16 June	1967	Loganair's first ambulance flight. Oronsay to Glasgow flown by Ken Foster in a Piper Aztec.
July	1967	First Britten-Norman Islander delivered to Loganair.
1 November	1971	BEA Helicopters begin SAR contract at Aberdeen for HM Coastguard.
6 December	1971	Eric Starling flies his last flight before retirement, an ambulance flight from Islay to Glasgow.
	1972	North Scottish Helicopters formed. Later to become Bond Helicopters.
1 April	1973	Full air ambulance service contract passes from BEA/British Airways to Loganair.
2 August	1973	Loganair's first inflight birth. Katy Devin born over Kirkwall en route to Aberdeen from Stronsay.
6 July	1988	Piper Alpha oil platform explosion.
20 December	1988	Pan-Am Boeing 747 disaster, Lockerbie.
2 April	1989	Kirsty Macleod born on HM Coastguard helicopter over Loch Erisort.
4 April	1989	Experimental ambulance helicopter service launched at Dundee in conjunction with Bond Helicopters and British Telecom.
1 February	1990	Experimental helicopter moves from Dundee to Inverness.
29 November	1990	Bond Helicopters' Bölkow BO 105D makes unscheduled stop on slopes of Meall Bac a' Choll Dhoire for birth of Mark Waugh.
April	1993	Contract awarded to Bond Helicopters to provide ambulance service using Bölkow BO 105D helicopters based at Prestwick and Inverness. Loganair to provide Islander aircraft in Orkney and Shetland.
15 November	1993	Loganair Islander, based at Glasgow, re-introduced to air ambulance service.

Appendix 3
Air Ambulance Aircraft

Air ambulance fixed-wing aircraft and helicopters have come in a wide variety of guises over six decades. This appendix provides details of some of the machines which have been used for air ambulance work on both a regular and occasional basis. The specifications given are for guidance only, detailed technical data being beyond the scope of this volume.

De Havilland DH84 Dragon	1933-1948	De Havilland DH60G Gipsy Moth	1947-1948
De Havilland DH80A Puss Moth	c1934-1939	Spartan Cruiser	1936-1940
De Havilland DH89		De Havilland DH114 Heron	1955-1973
Dragon Rapide	1936-1955	Britten-Norman BN-2 Islander	1967-
Piper Aztec PA23 250C	1967-1972	De Havilland Canada DHC-6	
Beech E18S	1968-1975	Twin Otter	1977-
Beechcraft Super King Air B200	1993-	Bölkow BO 105D	1989-
Aérospatiale Dauphin	1993-	Westland Dragonfly	1952-1967
Westland Whirlwind	1955-1981	Westland Wessex	1963-
Westland Sea King	1971-	Sikorsky S61N	1971-

De Havilland DH84 Dragon

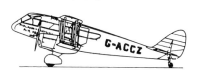

Powered by : Two de Havilland Gipsy Major I 4-cylinder 130hp inverted inline engines

Wingspan : 14.44 meters

Length : 10.52 meters

Cruising Speed: 109 mph, 175 kph

Range : 400 miles, 644 km

The first air ambulance flight was undertaken by Midland & Scottish Air Ferries' Dragon G-ACCZ from Islay to Renfrew on 14th May 1933 under the command of Captain Jimmy Orrell.

De Havilland Dragons were also used for air ambulance flights by Highland Airways, Northern & Scottish Airways, and Aberdeen Airways.

G-ACIT, formerly of Highland Airways, performed its last ambulance flight in 1948 before disposal by British European Airways. Edmund Fresson had wished to acquire the aircraft to operate a private ambulance service but BEA refused to consider sale of the aircraft to him. It is now based at Wroughton where it is in the care of the Science Museum.

De Havilland DH60G Gipsy Moth

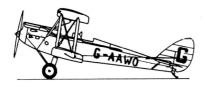

Powered by : One de Havilland
Gipsy I 85hp engine

Wingspan : 9.15 meters

Length : 7.29 meters

Cruising Speed: 85 mph, 137 kph

Range : 320 miles, 515 km

With two open cockpits and room for just one passenger, Edmund Fresson used the Gipsy Moth G-AAWO, built in 1930, for his first surveys of his planned operations in the north of Scotland.

The aircraft was pressed into service for air ambulance duties in the Orkney Islands upon several occasions during 1947 and 1948 by which time the new BEA had cut back on the operations of its predecessor in the Northern isles.

When Fresson parted company with BEA in March 1948 he was allowed to retain this aircraft but it was put up for sale later that year when he moved overseas. G-AAWO continues to fly in private ownership in the 1990s.

De Havilland DH80A Puss Moth

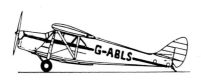

Powered by : One Gipsy III 120hp
inverted inline engine.

Wingspan : 11.21 meters

Length : 7.63 meters

Cruising Speed: 108 mph, 174 kph

Range : 300 miles, 483 km

Aberdeen Airways' DH80A Puss Moth G-ABLS is believed to have performed ambulance flights on several occasions. The aircraft was one of Eric Gandar Dower's personal collection which had flown in the King's Cup Race each year from 1931 until 1934. Following Gandar Dower's inauguration of Aberdeen Airways it frequently flew in support of the larger 'line' aircraft. On one ambulance flight, it operated from Aberdeen to Harrogate, not carrying a patient to hospital, but transporting a specialist to the aid of a patient. In the 1990s G-ABLS continued to fly in private ownership.

Spartan Cruiser

Powered by	: Three de Havilland Gipsy Major in-line piston engines (130hp)
Wingspan	: 16.47 meters
Length	: Mk. II 10.42 meters; Mk. III 12.50 meters
Cruising Speed:	115 mph, 185 kph
Max Range	: Mk. II 650 miles, 1,046 km; Mk. III 550 miles, 885 km

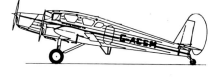

A total of seven Spartan Cruisers passed through the hands of Northern and Scottish Airways, five of these continuing in the service of its successor, Scottish Airways.

These were: Spartan Cruiser Mk. II G-ACSM, G-ACVT, G-ACYL and G-ACZM Spartan Cruiser Mk. III G-ACYK, G-ADEL and G-ADEM

Spartan Cruiser Mk. IIs were regularly used for ambulance flights until they were requisitioned by the RAF in 1940. (G-ACVT was written off after crashing at Glenbrittle Aerodrome, Skye, on 25th July 1936.)

Against a log entry for a Renfrew-Campbeltown-Islay return run on 4th November 1937, flown in Spartan Cruiser Mk. III G-ACYK, Captain David Barclay noted 'Pride of the Fleet'. On 15th January 1938 his log notes 'Search for YK'. G-ACYK had crashed on the Hill of Stake, Renfrewshire, the previous day. The shell of its fuselage, now at the Museum of Flight, East Fortune, is the only surviving reminder of the Spartan Cruiser.

De Havilland DH89 Dragon Rapide

Powered by	: Two 200hp de Havilland Gipsy VI 6-cylinder inverted inline air-cooled engines
Wingspan	: 14.64 meters
Length	: 10.52 meters
Cruising Speed	: 132 mph, 213 kph
Max Range	: 560 miles, 902 km

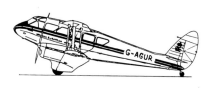

The DH89 Dragon Rapide was a 'souped up' Dragon with improved range, speed and payload. Northern & Scottish Airways, Highland Airways and Aberdeen Airways all added Rapides to their fleets during the mid-1930s. Good performance with one engine closed down gave added confidence to operators traversing wide stretches of open water.

Upon the formation of BEA, the Rapide, which the state corporation called the 'Islander' class, was the mainstay of its ambulance service. David Barclay flew BEA's last Rapide flight in Scotland, in G-AHKS, to collect a patient from Campbeltown, on 28th May 1955.

De Havilland DH114 Heron 1B

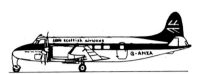

Powered by	: Four 250hp de Havilland Gipsy Queen 30 Mk.2 piston engines
Wingspan	: 21.81 meters
Length	: 14.79 meters
Cruising Speed:	183 mph, 295 kph
Range	: 1,180 miles, 1900 km

British European Airways employed three Herons, which it called the 'Hebrides' class, on ambulance duties between 1955 and 1973.

G-ANXA First named *John Hunter*. Hunter (1728-1793) was born at Long Calderwood, Lanarkshire, and was a pioneer in pathological anatomy. G-ANXA was later renamed *Sister Jean Kennedy* after the nurse who was killed when sister ship G-AOFY crashed on Islay in 1957.

G-ANXB *Sir James Young Simpson*. Simpson (1811-1870) was born in Bathgate. His innovations included the introduction of chloroform as a general anaesthetic.

G-AOFY *Sir Charles Bell*. Bell (1774-1842) was born in Edinburgh. A distinguished anatomist, he did much pioneering research into the workings of the nervous system. On 28th September 1957 G-AOFY was destroyed in the fatal crash on Islay.

Piper PA23-250C Aztec

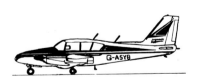

Powered by	: Two 250hp Lycoming piston engines
Wingspan	: 11.34m
Length	: 9.52m
Cruising Speed:	210 mph, 338 kph
Range	: 1,210 miles, 1,947 km

Loganair operated its first ambulance flight on 16th June 1967 when G-ASYB conveyed a patient from Oronsay to Glasgow.

Between 1962 and 1972 Loganair operated four Aztec aircraft. PA23-250A (G-ARMH), PA23-250B (G-ASER and G-ASNA), PA23-250C (G-ASYB). Only G-ASYB, delivered in 1964, was still in the fleet when Loganair undertook its first air ambulance contract.

Britten-Norman BN-2 Islander

Powered by   : Two 260hp Avco
Lycoming piston
engines (BN-2A)
Wingspan   : 14.94m
Length   : 10.86m
Cruising Speed: 158 mph, 254 kph
Range   : 800 miles, 1,287 km

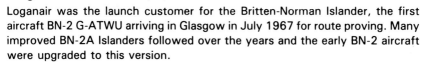

Loganair was the launch customer for the Britten-Norman Islander, the first aircraft BN-2 G-ATWU arriving in Glasgow in July 1967 for route proving. Many improved BN-2A Islanders followed over the years and the early BN-2 aircraft were upgraded to this version.

The names *Sir James Young Simpson, Sister Jean Kennedy, Captain David Barclay MBE OStJ, Captain F E Fresson OBE, E L Gandar Dower Esq, Robert McKean OBE FCIT,* and *Captain Eric A Starling FRMetS* have appeared upon different occasions on many of Loganair's Islanders.

Pilatus Britten-Norman BN2B aircraft operated by Loganair appeared in the colour scheme of the Scottish Ambulance Service in 1993.

Beech E18S

Powered by   : Two 450hp Pratt &
Whitney radial piston
engines
Wingspan   : 15.14 meters
Length   : 10.73 meters
Cruising Speed: 185 mph 298 kph
Range   : 1,530 miles 2,462km

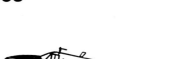

The prototype of the American-built Beech 18 was flown in 1937. Over 9,000 aircraft of all variants of the type were built until production finally came to a close in the 1970s.

Loganair operated Beech E18S G-ASUG from 1968 until 1975. The aircraft was acquired by the airline for its long range capability to use on its first international service which linked Scotland with Bergen. But the aircraft was used in many other roles which included executive air charters.

It was a natural aircraft for longer distance ambulance flights, such as those to carry transplant patients to specialist hospitals in the south of England, and it was used on numerous occasions on ambulance flights within Scotland. G-ASUG is now on display at the Museum of Flight, East Fortune.

De Havilland Canada DHC-6-300 Twin Otter

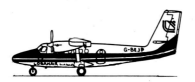

Powered by	: Two 652 eshp Pratt & Whitney PT6A-27 turboprop engines
Wingspan	: 19.81 meters
Length	: 15.77 meters
Cruising Speed:	210 mph, 338 kph
Range	: 1,103 miles, 1,775 km

Loganair frequently employed the Twin Otter on longer distance ambulance flights, most notably those transferring organ transplant patients to specialist hospitals in the south of England.

Loganair's first DHC-6 Twin Otter, G-BELS was delivered on 17th March 1977. Loganair continues to operate a Twin Otter, which can be seen in the livery of British Airways Express, on scheduled services to Tiree and Barra.

Beechcraft Super King Air B200

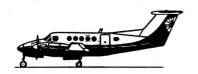

Powered by	: Two eshp Pratt & Whitney PT6A-42 turboprop engines
Wingspan	: 16.61m
Length	: 13.34m
Cruising Speed:	333 mph, 536 kph
Range	: 2,142 miles, 3,447 km

The Beechcraft Super King Air was introduced to the Scottish Air Ambulance Service in 1993 with the awarding of a contract to Bond Aviation.

The Super King Air plays a supplementary role to the Bölkow BO 105D helicopters also supplied by Bond, and is operated on an occasional basis as the need arises. From its Aberdeen base the Super King Air can reach Kirkwall or Glasgow in 30 minutes, Stornoway in 40 minutes and Sumburgh in 50 minutes.

Its speed makes it especially attractive for carrying transplant patients requiring to be moved over longer distances necessary to reach hospitals specialising in such surgery in England. Loganair operated a Beech E18S in a similar role between 1968 and 1975.

Bölkow BO 105D

Powered by : Two Allison
250-C20B turbine
engines
Rotor Diameter: 9.84 meters
Length : 8.58 meters
Cruising Speed: 140mph, 225kph
Range : 340 miles, 547 km

The Bölkow BO 105D, manufactured by Messerschmit-Bölkow-Blohm GmbH of Munich, was first used for the Scottish Air Ambulance Service when G-BATC was based at Dundee Airport in 1989.

Operated by Bond Helicopters Ltd for the Scottish Ambulance Service, G-BATC was initially operated for a six-month trial with major sponsorship provided by British Telecom. The trial was extended for a further six-month period during which G-BATC was relocated to Inverness.

With the awarding of a contract to Bond Helicopters in 1993 to provide air ambulance cover for the Scottish Ambulance Service, two Bölkow BO 105Ds were provided, one based at Inverness and the other at Prestwick.

The Air Support Unit of Strathclyde Police has operated a Bölkow BO 105 since November 1989. Fitted with a stretcher facility, it is tasked occasionally for casevac cases in life-threatening situations.

Aérospatiale Dauphin

Powered by : Two Turbomeca
Arriel 630 shp
turboshafts

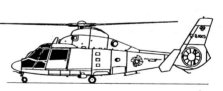

Rotor diameter: 11.68m
Length : 11.00m
Max Speed : 196 mph, 315 kph
Range : 283 miles, 455 km

The Aérospatiale SA 365C Dauphin of Bond Helicopters' base at Plockton came into the service of the Scottish Ambulance Service from April 1993. The Dauphin is not a dedicated aircraft to the ambulance service but can operate ambulance flights on an 'as available' basis.

In this role it is a useful back-up to the operator's Bölkow BO 105D helicopters with its greater speed and carrying capacity. The Dauphin came into service in 1977 and can operate with a crew of two pilots, a winchman, and a winch operator. It can carry two stretchers or ten seated patients.

Westland Dragonfly

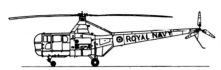

Powered by : Alvis Leonides 50
520hp
Rotor Diameter: 14.94m
Length : 12.53m
Cruising Speed: 85mph, 137kph
Range : 248 miles, 400 km

The Westland Dragonfly was first stationed at Lossiemouth by the Royal Navy in 1952. Described as the Royal Navy's first 'real helicopter', it marked the transition by the Search and Rescue services from fixed-wing amphibious aircraft to the helicopter age.

Westland Whirlwind

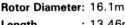

Powered by : Bristol Siddeley
Gnome H.1000
1,050shp turboshafts
Rotor Diameter: 16.1m
Length : 13.46m
Max Speed : 106mph, 170kph
Range : 300 miles, 483 km

The Westland Whirlwind was a version of the American-built Sikorsky S-55, constructed under licence. It was first employed in a Search and Rescue role in 1955 and continued in various upgraded forms until 1981, latterly as the HAR Mk 9 with the Royal Navy and the HAR Mk 10 with the RAF.

Westland Wessex

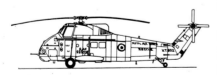

Powered by : Two Rolls-Royce
1,350shp turboshafts
Rotor Diameter: 17.08 meters
Length : 15.10 meters
Max Speed : 152mph, 245kph
Range : 478 miles, 770km

Built by Westland under licence from Sikorsky, which designated their version as the Sikorsky S-58, the Wessex has had a long career in Search and Rescue with both the Royal Navy and the Royal Air Force.

Operating with a crew of four, the Wessex can carry up to sixteen survivors. The Royal Navy operated the Wessex from 1963 until 1988. The RAF expects to retire its Wessex aircraft during the mid-1990s.

Westland Sea King

Powered by   : Two 1.238kW (1,660shp)
                     Rolls Royce Gnome
                     H.1400-1 turboshafts

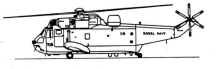

Rotor diameter : 18.9m
Length   : 17.01m
Max Speed   : 129 mph, 207 kph
Range   : 765 miles, 1,230 km

The Westland Sea King is a development of the Sikorsky S-61 and is widely employed both by the Royal Navy at Prestwick and by the RAF at Lossiemouth and Boulmer for Search and Rescue work.

When 819 Squadron of the Royal Navy arrived at Prestwick in 1971 it came equipped with the Sea King Mark 1. 819 Squadron has worked through various upgradings of the aircraft, taking delivery of the Mark 5 in 1985 and Mark 6 in 1989. D Flight of 202 Squadron RAF at Lossiemouth took delivery of its first Sea King in September 1978. The Sea King also served with D Flight of 22 Squadron RAF at Leuchars.

While participating in a Mountain Rescue training exercise from RAF Lossiemouth on 28th January 1989, Sea King Mark 3, XV585. crashed on 3,700' Creag Meagaidh in the southern Monadhliath Mountains, after an engine failed. All of the occupants survived without major injury.

Sikorsky S61N

Powered by   : Two 1,500shp General
                      Electric CT58-140-2
                      turboshaft engines
Rotor Diameter : 18.9 meters
Length   : 17.96 meters
Cruising Speed : 138mph, 222kph
Range   : 518 miles, 833 km

Cousin to the Sea King, the Sikorsky S61N was certified in 1964, and flew in a SAR role with BEA Helicopters on contract to HM Coastguard at Aberdeen from 1971. This continued until 1983 by which time the contract had moved from Aberdeen to Sumburgh (1979). Bristow Helicopters then took over the Coastguard contract at Sumburgh, again flying the Sikorsky S61N, and in 1987 a second S61N was based at Stornoway.

In 1988 the Stornoway S61N crashed into the sea while hovering at low altitude during a search for missing fishermen. A Sea King from RAF Lossiemouth uplifted the ditched aircrew. A fragment of rotor blade from the unfortunate S61N now adorns the wall of the Bristow crew room at Stornoway.

The specially equipped SAR helicopters of Bristow which currently operate the HM Coastguard contracts are G-BIMU at Stornoway and G-BDOC at Sumburgh.

Acknowledgements

A compilation of this nature would not have been possible without the help, co-operation, and enthusiasm of a large number of people. I would particularly like to thank Nurse Margaret Boyd, now a youthful 90 year old; Tony Naylor, former Operations Manager of B.E.A. at Glasgow; Scott Grier, Managing Director of Loganair; and Captain Ken Foster, former Operations Director of Loganair. Special thanks are due to my good friend Ron Davies who kindly wrote the foreword and gave much valuable advice on the manuscript. And to Captain David Dyer who, in addition to offering regular encouragement, arranged first-hand experience of travel on the flight-deck of an air ambulance Islander.

Additionally I would like to thank the following from the world of aviation: Captain Andy Alsop; Captain Roger Asbey; Captain Ben Bamber; Captain Peter Black; Captain Mike Bond; Steve Branley; Captain Ken Browning; Catherine Cameron (née MacGeachy); Gilbert Carswell; John Corrigan; Linda Doak; Flt Lt J I Gilchrist; Captain Phil Green; Captain Vivian Gunton; David L Hall; Captain Don Hoare; Tab Hunter; Captain Arthur Kerr; Alex Knight; Craig Lindsay; Jack Long; Alex Macarthur; Coll Macdonald; Captain Jim McDonald; Captain Kenneth McLean; Captain David Marris; Captain Ian Montgomery; Captain Geoff Northmore; Captain Mike O'Brien; Bill Palmer; Lt Angus Paterson; Ronald Philpot; Brian Piket; Harry S Robert; Tom B Siddell; Captain Eric Starling; Lt Neill Stephenson, Flt Lt Nick Stillwell; Captain George Stone; Captain Henry Vallance, Lt Jon Webster, Captain Alan Whitfield; Iain Winnard; Captain Nick Wright; Captain Tom Wright.

From the medical profession: Irene Barr; Ellen Buchanan (née Hutchison); Dr Alex M Campbell; Derek W Card; Lesley Crawford; Robert Devine; Elisabeth Douglas; Andy Fuller; Ian Golding; Miss E M Inglis; Steve Jelfs; Gerry Kelly; Mike Knell; John Lyall; Dr John A J Macleod; Dr Robert J Martin; Christina Ann Morrison (née MacRitchie); June Neil; Islay Skea; John West.

Thanks are due also to: Jonathan Ayres; Margaret Ayres; Peter Clegg; Maureen Clyne; G S Cook; Rev John R H Cormack; The Courier and Advertiser; Alistair Goldsmith, University of Strathclyde; Alistair Gordon of The Orcadian; Elaine Hamilton; Sheila Harper (née Barclay); Wendy Johnson; Alick Macaulay; Donald Macaulay; David McCallum; David McIntosh; Laurence Macintyre, Strathclyde Police; Duncan Macmillan; Catrìona McPhee; Jean Muir; the staff of the Museum of Islay Life, Port Charlotte; Ian Purvis; Simon Riley, HM Coastguard; Muriel Robertson; Ronnie Rodger; Chief Superintendent Mel Strachan, Strathclyde Police; Helen McCaig Sutton (née Reid); Woman Magazine.

The paintings of Scottish Ambulance Service Islander aircraft G-BPCA over the Isle of Tiree were kindly produced by aviation artist Colin Taylor. When not painting, Colin is to be found on the flightdeck of one of the Shorts 360 aircraft of Loganair with whom he has been flying since 1989. Chris Weir has given encouragement and support over the years and has continued to do so in guiding the evolution of this story from manuscript to book.

Finally, I would again like to thank Chuti, Panee, and Narin for their forbearance over the months during which this project was coming together.

Bibliography

Aviation in Scotland.   J D Gillies and J L Wood
Glasgow Branch of the Royal Aeronautical Society 1966

Air Road to the Isles   Captain E.E. Fresson
Published by David Rendal 1967

Lifeline to the Islands   Robert McKean OBE FC InstT
British European Airways 1973

Scottish Air Mails   Richard Beith
Published by Richard Beith, Chester, 1981

Pleunaichean na Gàidhealtachd   Ruairidh MacLeòid
Crùisgean, Loch nam Madadh (Lochmaddy), 1982

1000 Up   A B Clancey and A J Wright
BN Historians, Staines, 1983

Guide to the Aircraft Collection C L Thompson and J D Storer
Royal Scottish Museum 1983

A Flying Start to the Day   Peter V Clegg
Published by Peter V Clegg 1986

Flying against the Elements   Peter V Clegg
Published by Peter V Clegg 1987

The Story of Loganair   Iain Hutchison
Western Isles Publishing Co Ltd, Stornoway, 1987

Railway Air Services   John Stroud
Ian Allan Ltd, Shepperton, 1987

An Illustrated History of British European Airways Phil Lo Bao
Browcom Group plc, Feltham, 1989

Glasgow's Airport   Dugald Cameron
Holmes McDougall Ltd, Edinburgh, 1990

Sword in the Sky   Peter V Clegg
Published by Peter V Clegg 1990

Rescue   Paul Beaver and Paul Berriff
Patrick Stephens Ltd, Wellingborough, 1990

For Those in Peril — 50 Years of Royal Navy Search and Rescue John Winton
Robert Hale, London, 1992

The Flight of the Starling — Iain Hutchison
Kea Publishing, Erskine, 1992

HMS Gannet — The Story So Far — E J Buckett, T W Bishop and I G Armstrong
Published privately 1993

Wings over the Glens — Peter V Clegg
GMS Enterprises, Peterborough, 1995

Island Pilot — Alan Whitfield
The Shetland Times Ltd, Lerwick, 1995

By the same Author
Two unique perspectives of the Scottish Aviation Story

The Flight of the Starling

The flying career of Scottish pioneer aviator Captain Eric Starling
'A nice book and very heavily illustrated'
Jimmie MacGregor, BBC Radio Scotland.
'A super read ... a story of Scotland; a story of the changes in Scotland'
Alex Dickson, Radio Clyde.
Published in 1992 by Kea Publishing, Erskine
ISBN 09518958 0 X
Price £9.95

The Story of Loganair

Scotland's Airline, the first 25 years
'A most readable book, well produced and one of the most useful volumes to cross my desk for some time past'
J D Ferguson, Aviation News
'Will appeal to the aviation enthusiast and general reader alike with its lively and informative style'
Business and Finance
Published in 1987 by Western Isles Publishing Co. Ltd, Stornoway
ISBN 0906437 14 8
Price £4.95

Both titles available from:
Kea Publishing, 14 Flures Crescent, Erskine, Renfrewshire, PA8 7DJ, Scotland
(Please add 10% UK, 15% Overseas Surface, 25% Overseas Airmail)